W9-CLO-183

THE
KINESIOLOGY
WORKBOOK

Second Edition

THE KINESIOLOGY WORKBOOK

Second Edition

Jan F. Perry, EdD, PT
Professor and Chairman
Department of Physical Therapy
School of Allied Health Sciences
Medical College of Georgia
Augusta, Georgia

David A. Rohe, MPH, PT
Adjunct Assistant Professor
Department of Physical Therapy
School of Allied Health Sciences
Medical College of Georgia
Augusta, Georgia
and
Clinical Director
Ginger Hill Clinic
Thomson, Georgia

Anita O. Garcia, MS, PT
Harker Heights, Texas

F. A. DAVIS COMPANY • Philadelphia

F. A. Davis Company
1915 Arch Street
Philadelphia, PA 19103

Printed in the United States of America

Last digit indicates print number: 10 9 8 7

Publisher: Jean-François Vilain
Developmental Editor: Crystal McNichol
Production Editor: Jessica Howie Martin
Cover Designer: Louis Forgione

As new scientific information becomes available through basic and clinical research, recommended treatments and drug therapies undergo changes. The authors and publisher have done everything possible to make this book accurate, up to date, and in accord with accepted standards at the time of publication. The authors, editors, and publisher are not responsible for errors or omissions or for consequences from application of the book, and make no warranty, expressed or implied, in regard to the contents of the book. Any practice described in this book should be applied by the reader in accordance with professional standards of care used in regard to the unique circumstances that may apply in each situation. The reader is advised always to check product information (package inserts) for changes and new information regarding dose and contraindications before administering any drug. Caution is especially urged when using new or infrequently ordered drugs.

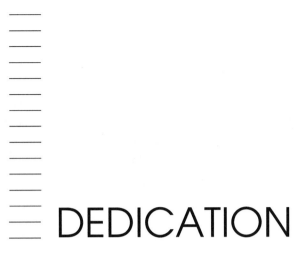

DEDICATION

For the many weekends, early mornings, and late evenings given up, we wish to thank our children—Vince, Erin, Hannah, and Sarah.

For the tasks left to them to handle (children, dishes, meals, and moral support), we wish to thank our spouses—Bob and Sharon.

For all of those who are committed to a process of learning that blurs the difference between learners and teachers, we are most thankful.

PREFACE TO THE SECOND EDITION

Over the past 4 years, we have been using this workbook in our physical therapy program. In that time, our students have pointed out what they liked, some dilemmas, and some errors. They have asked insightful questions about some of the items and some of the answers. They, and our colleagues across the country and *their* students, have challenged us. We have found activities that were difficult for students to understand and activities that were highly effective in facilitating learning. Mostly, however, we have been convinced of the value of having students manipulate information and struggle with difficult concepts.

In this revision, we have addressed many of the issues that have been raised about the workbook. The former first chapter has been divided into two—one chapter dealing solely with biomechanics and the other with concepts related to patient evaluation. Other chapters have had terminology updated, unclear items or answers clarified, new activities added, errors corrected, and ineffective activities eliminated.

The basic philosophy and purpose of *The Kinesiology Workbook,* second edition, continues to be one of providing students with the opportunity to wrestle with difficult concepts and to manipulate information. Let us hear from you about your uses of the workbook.

JFP
DAR
AOG

PREFACE TO THE FIRST EDITION

The Kinesiology Workbook has evolved over many years of teaching an introductory physical therapy course on the basics of patient evaluation—kinesiology, goniometry, and muscle testing. We developed this book to help our students bridge the gap between the textbook presentations of these subjects and the actual physical assessment of *normal* movement—the gap between knowing and doing.

Briefly, *The Kinesiology Workbook* offers an array of exercises related to general principles of kinesiology and biomechanics, to each major joint, and to gait and posture evaluation. The exercises include both homework and classwork, and consist of both individual and group activities.

Our teaching, and therefore this book, is based on the assumption that the manipulation of data and concepts enhances learning. Some of the manipulations in *The Kinesiology Workbook* are physical, while others are mental. All the exercises are designed to encourage students to make connections between what they have read and what they will be doing in the clinical setting.

This workbook will be of value to students in physical therapy, occupational therapy, athletic training, exercise science, exercise physiology, and physical education. It can be used to supplement introductory texts in kinesiology, functional anatomy, and gross anatomy. As educators, we know that different people learn in different ways, so we encourage students and teachers to choose the exercises most useful to them, to adapt any that can be made more useful, and to skip those that do not apply to their learning situation. For example, drawing the muscles and completing outlines enhances learning for some students but not for others. Those for whom drawing the muscles is helpful can complete the charts, while the others go on to different exercises.

The key to *The Kinesiology Workbook* is that it is designed to be *used,* not merely to be read. We would appreciate hearing from you about your successes and problems in using *The Kinesiology Workbook* and about any successful adaptations of the exercises that you have used.

JFP
DAR
AOG

ACKNOWLEDGMENTS FOR THE SECOND EDITION

We wish to thank Jeff Dowling for his input into the revision of the chapter on the foot and ankle. His work in that area has served to strengthen that chapter.

Doug Keskula has joined our teaching team and has enhanced the workbook by giving us another point of view.

Without a doubt, our students are our greatest teachers. The classes of 1993 through 1996 have been unstinting in their comments about the workbook. Their contributions are responsible for most of the changes in the workbook.

Editorial encouragement has been consistently provided by Jean-François Vilain. We have appreciated his wit, his persistence, and his hospitality.

ACKNOWLEDGMENTS FOR THE FIRST EDITION

Active engagement of the learner is a cornerstone of the teaching style that initiated the development of this book. For that philosophical orientation we thank Drs. Carl Rogers and Jerome Bruner. For the curriculum that has allowed us to practice that philosophy, we thank Bella J. May, EdD, PT.

Many people were involved with the development of the kinesiology course for which this book was originally written. We would like to take this opportunity to express our appreciation to Dennis Hart, Rita DeFazio, Cathy Koshman, Ann Charness, Donna Zorn, and Harold Smith.

For editorial assistance in the original draft of this book, we wish to thank Sandra Eskew Capps.

Karen Waldo, David Mascaro, and Milton Burroughs in the Department of Medical Illustration and Design of the Medical College of Georgia are responsible for the fine illustrations in this book. Their work speaks for itself.

We are thankful for the assistance provided by the following reviewers: Phyllis L. Beck, MEd, PT; Leonard Elbaum, PT; Alta J. Hansen, PhD, PT; Carolyn Kisner, MS, PT; Cynthia C. Norkin, EdD, PT; M. Lynn Palmer, PhD, PT; Thomas J. Schmitz, MS, PT; and D. Joyce White, MS, PT.

In addition to the contributions cited above, the students who have participated in our classes have given us invaluable feedback. Physical Therapy classes of the Medical College of Georgia from 1981–1992, we thank you.

CONTENTS

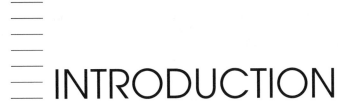

INTRODUCTION

The study of the functioning of the human body is intriguing and challenging. The concepts and information in the field of kinesiology and applied anatomy are highly physical and manipulative, but textbooks tend to be theoretical and cognitive. This workbook provides an opportunity to use the information in your texts in a physical and manipulative manner. You will be applying information that you gain from other sources, often bringing information from several sources together. The act of bringing together information from many sources to apply to a problem is directly applicable to the way you will be functioning once you graduate. Practical problems, such as those found in the clinic, require practical solutions rather than recitation.

The major purpose of this book is to provide you with the opportunity to apply information. We have purposely avoided presenting information in this book. Many sources already exist to provide sound kinesiological and applied anatomy information. We assume that you will use those sources to gather the information needed to solve the problems and aid in the activities presented here.

Another purpose of this workbook is to provide activities that will help you begin to develop your skills in exercise design. Many of the activities will have you determine how to create an exercise or motion or to obtain a position to accomplish a specific purpose. This is similar to designing a specific exercise to accomplish a patient or client goal. Several activities in this workbook are designed to reinforce goniometry and muscle-testing *principles*. We have not attemped to provide a goniometry or muscle-testing text.

Chapter 1 asks you to apply general principles of biomechanics. Chapter 2 is related to basic principles of kinesiology. Many of these principles are directly related to the basic patient-client evaluation skills of muscle testing, goniometry, and palpation. Chapters 3 through 10 are related to body segments or major joints of the body. Chapter 3 addresses the complex functioning of the spine and pelvis. Chapters 4, 5, and 6 progress through the lower extremities: hip, knee, and foot and ankle, respectively. Chapters 7 through 9 relate to the upper extremities. Chapter 7 details the functioning of the shoulder complex. The elbow is presented in Chapter 8, and the wrist and hand are the topics of Chapter 9. Chapter 10 presents the temporomandibular joint complex. Chapters 11 and 12 deal with posture and gait, respectively. Generally, each chapter starts with less difficult information and builds to more complex information.

In this day of women's and men's liberation, the use of pronouns can become a major issue. We believe that "he/she" is awkward, that the sole use of the masculine pronoun is inappropriate, and that the text should be readable. Therefore, we have adopted a convention to deal with the gender pronouns—the odd-numbered chapters have the feminine pronoun and the even-numbered chapters have the masculine pronoun.

The greatest benefit will be derived from this book if you go through the described activities in a manner open to discovery. Trust that the activity will lead you to the appropriate information. Perform the activity, then explain what happened. Bring information to the activity from your anatomy and kinesiology texts. *Think* about what you have been asked to do or have done. The research and thinking that you do to complete the activity and the discussion following completion of the activity are critical to your learning. Answering the questions (filling in all of the blanks) is less important. Answers are provided at the end of each chapter to assist you in confirming your information. In our experience with students in our classes, going to the answers too quickly will allow you to fill in all the blanks in a timely manner; however, it will also markedly decrease your learning.

Some activities are paper-and-pencil questions; others are quite physical and require some equipment or props. We have marked with asterisks (*) those items that we consider more physical activities. These often require a partner, and sometimes a small group of fellow students.

Many of the activities in this workbook provide time to explore with your classmates. In many instances, you are asked to "design a method of measuring" something, "determine landmarks" to assess a motion, or "determine how to stretch" something. In many instances, there are standard ways of doing what is requested. In some activities, we have chosen not to provide those standards, but to let you choose whatever standards make sense to you and can be defended to your classmates and faculty. We believe that there is great value in determining a defensible method (to measure, assess, or stretch), based on your understanding of the anatomy and biomechanics involved in the situation. This does not negate the critical importance of standardized methods of measurement. Rather, it emphasizes the importance of understanding why the standards were chosen. That understanding will assist you in adapting standards when a patient's or client's needs demand something nonstandard.

Because of our belief in the discovery method of learning, some of the items in the workbook appear to be incomplete or lacking some information. This is done purposely to provide you with the opportunity to use your texts to solve problems as you would in the "real world."

As stated earlier, this workbook is not intended to stand without other texts; it requires other texts for information to use in completing the activities. This text is also best utilized with someone who has a strong clinical and kinesiological background. Some of the activities are best demonstrated by someone with such a background. Some of the discussions associated with items in the workbook need input from faculty or others with appropriate expertise (kinesiology, anatomy, biomechanics, and clinical practice). Do not hesitate to request clarification if it seems useful. Do not forget that your classmates are a rich source of information. In our physical therapy program, it is not uncommon to have students who are certified athletic trainers, exercise physiologists, or other individuals who have significant clinical experience to share with the class. Often the understanding of these classmates can do more to help others in the class learn a concept than additional explanation from the faculty. Talk to and learn from each other. We firmly believe that learning should be fun. Creating this workbook has been fun and a source of much learning. So, have fun as you jump into the study of how our bodies work!

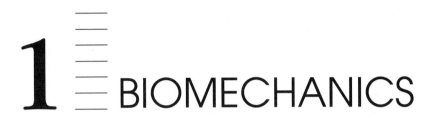

1 BIOMECHANICS

This chapter provides exercises and problems to help you understand some of the basic principles of kinematics and kinetics, that is, the definition and description of movements and the analysis of the forces influencing the movements. The earlier items in the chapter are easier and the later ones more difficult, building on the understanding derived from the earlier part of the chapter. You will need outside resources to answer the problems or perform the activities, which are grouped by concepts. We begin with kinematics.

NAMES OF MOVEMENTS

1. What do you call the *movement* when you are standing erect in the anatomical position and you:
   a. *Bend* your elbow from a fully straight to a 90° bent position? _____
   b. Maintain the 90° elbow bent position, but *turn* your palm down? _____
   c. Maintain the 90° elbow bent position, but *turn* your palm up? _____
   d. Maintain the 90° elbow bent position, keep your elbow touching your side, and *turn* your arm out so that your fingers are pointing directly away from your side? _____
   e. Maintain the 90° elbow bent position, keep your elbow touching your side, and *turn* your arm back so that your fingers are pointing directly forward? _____
   f. *Straighten* your elbow? _____
   g. *Move* your arm laterally away from your side until it is parallel to the floor?

   _____

   h. *Move* your arm back down to your side? _____

   The above movements are examples applied to your shoulder, elbow, and forearm. Similar illustrations can be applied to your wrist, hand, fingers, hip, knee, toes, and trunk. The movements in the ankle are typically named differently, as are some of the wrist and spinal movements.

2. Give the synonym(s) that you find used for ankle, spine, and wrist movements in the following list. Consult different texts such as your anatomy, kinesiology, goniometry, and muscle-testing texts for the synonyms.

   Ankle

   Dorsiflexion _____

   Plantarflexion _____

   Spine

   Flexion _____

Extension _____

Lateral flexion _____

Wrist

Radial deviation _____

Ulnar deviation _____

3. Name the *joint position* when your limb is placed as follows:

   a. Elbow bent to 90° _____

   b. Elbow straight _____

   c. Palm up as in 1c above _____

   d. Palm down as in 1b above _____

4. What is the name of the *movement* when:

   a. You straighten your elbow from the 90° bent position to the 45° bent position?

   b. You bring your arm down from a position of straight out to the side at shoulder height to a position 45° out to the side?

   c. From a position of reaching as far as you can behind you, you bring your arm forward until your hand is just slightly behind your hip, keeping your elbow straight?

   The point that is being made here is that your language must be clear as to whether you are describing a movement (action) or a position. The same root words can be used for positions and actions, and actions must be clearly described in order to avoid miscommunication.

5. A method of specifying joint motions is the Rule of Three (McKeough, DM, unpublished monograph). In using the Rule of Three, one names the movement, the bone or part that is moving, and the joint at which motion is occurring. This is in contrast to the more common method of naming motions by just movement and joint. Using this rule, item 1a would be called flexion of the forearm at the elbow rather than flexion of the elbow; 1d would be lateral rotation of the humerus at the shoulder rather than lateral rotation of the shoulder. The usefulness of this rule will be more apparent when we discuss reverse actions in Chapter 2. Below, develop a full list of voluntary movements available at the shoulder and the knee, but using the clearer terminology found in the Rule of Three.

*6. In order to move ourselves or objects in space, the angular motion that occurs around our joints must become linear motion. Observe a subject and describe the angular motion that occurs in each of the following bones to accomplish the described actions:

   a. Humerus at the shoulder and forearm at the elbow to push a book away from the body across the surface of a table.

   b. Femur at the hip and tibia at the knee to pull a book across the floor from in front to under the subject. This is best illustrated if the subject is seated.

PLANES AND AXES

7. What is another name for the coronal plane? _____

8. What is another name for the horizontal plane? _____

*9. Use a stiff piece of paper such as the back of a tablet and place it parallel to each of the cardinal planes of your body or your partner's body. This activity is to provide you with a physical representation of the imaginary two-dimensional cardinal planes. For a pictorial representation of these planes, see the diagrams in Chapter 3.

*10. A way to visualize an axis is to use a pencil or other straight object that produces a straight line. Place the pencil pointing at the shoulder so that if it went through the shoulder joint, you could visualize the humerus turning on it. The pencil would be a turning point for the humerus at the shoulder. Now, with the shoulder starting in the anatomical position for each movement below, place the pencil so that the humerus turns to produce:

   a. Flexion and extension
   b. Adduction and abduction
   c. Medial and lateral rotation

11. Name the plane and axis for each motion in 10 above. For our purposes, an axis will be named by the direction of its orientation, that is, medial-lateral, anterior-posterior, vertical.

                   Plane   **Axis**

   a. _____ and _____

   b. _____ and _____

   c. _____ and _____

12. Give the planes in which the following motions take place. (For our purposes of naming movements, the planes will be named in relation to the body. Note that in dissection or surgery, the plane of the particular view or cut is in relation to the part studied assuming anatomical position. We are studying movement and want the plane of the movement in relation to the subject's body.)

   a. Stepping up a step _____

   b. Side step with the right leg (movement of the stepping leg) _____

   c. Turning a screwdriver with the forearm:

       As in 1c above _____

       With forearm at the side _____

   d. Shaking head "no" _____

   e. Straight sit-up _____

   f. Side bending of the trunk _____

BASE OF SUPPORT

*13. Take the ink barrel out of the pen you are using (assuming you are using a ballpoint pen) and stand the empty holder on the tapered end. It should stand alone. Repeat the procedure with the ink barrel back in the pen, standing it on the point. Explain the difference in result using the principles of line of gravity and base of support.

*14. Apply this activity to yourself in standing. What would you do to demonstrate the effect of a diminished base of support?

*15. Now apply the principle in the hands-and-knees position. What does your body do when one of the four sources of support is removed?

CENTER OF MASS/LINE OF GRAVITY

*16. Find the point where the composite center of mass is located in your pen or pencil.

  a. How did you do it? How could you find it in a classmate?

  b. Now define center of mass.

*17. For the activities in this item, you will need a plumb line, additional string, a tongue depressor, tape, stickers labeled A and B, and a subject in laboratory clothes.

  a. Ask the subject to stand, and place a stick-on marker labeled A on the lateral aspect of the body lateral to where the body's composite center of mass is considered to be located. Drop a plumb line from the marker. Where does the line fall in relation to the feet?

  b. Have the subject sit on a stool. When the subject is sitting, the center of mass has moved to a point on the anterior surface of the body just above the navel (approximately). Put a second marker B on the subject lateral to this point. Drop a plumb line from this point. Where does the line fall in relation to the feet?

  c. Ask the subject to *slowly* come to a standing position with no trunk or hip flexion. Record what happens to the subject. Did sticker B ever appear to be over the feet?

  d. Now allow trunk and hip flexion and ask the subject to repeat the activity. Be sure the subject moves slowly in order to watch the alignment of sticker B in relation to the feet. At the point when the subject first begins to rise, stop the movement and record where the plumb line from B falls relative to the position of the feet. When the subject first begins to rise, where are the subject's head and shoulders in relation to the feet?

    HINT: Attach a weighted string to the lateral side of the subject's shoulder so the string extends out to the side and the weight falls to the side of the seat. A tongue depressor taped to the top of the shoulder with the string hanging down from it usually works.

Discuss your findings in terms of:

- Shift in line of gravity of the trunk
- Relationship between the line of gravity and the base of support in coming to stand
- How this activity relates to item 13

EFFECTS OF GRAVITY

*18. For the three activities listed below, decide what force is the prime mover for the action, what muscles are active during the action, and what type of contraction (concentric, eccentric, isometric) the muscles are performing. When identifying the responsible muscles, use groupings such as flexors, extensors, or abductors of the joint(s) in question rather than muscle names. Perform the action or have a partner perform the action and palpate the muscles to verify your observations.

While standing, perform the indicated actions:

a. Slowly *lower* a 10-lb weight from the flexed elbow to the fully extended elbow position.

b. Slowly *bend* forward at the waist.

c. Stand on your right leg and pick up the left foot. Hold onto a table for balance and slowly *flex* your *right* knee from the fully extended position.

Remember that you are concentrating on the movement, not the new position assumed.

19. In item 18 the movements performed were extension of the forearm at the elbow, flexion of the trunk and pelvis at the hip, and flexion of the femur and the tibia at the knee. The muscle groups that are usually the prime movers for these actions are, of course, the elbow extensors, trunk and hip flexors, and knee flexors, respectively. Explain to your landlady, who is unfamiliar with kinesiology, why these muscles were not needed in the actions as performed.

*

20. Now do the following:

a. Place your body or limb in a position for each of the movements in item 18 so that the movement is caused by the muscle group responsible for the action; that is, the elbow extensors cause extension of the forearm at the elbow, and so on. Make sure your positioning does not allow gravity to assist with the movement.

b. Record the position of the limb or your body that satisfied the criteria.

c. What type of contraction was performed by the muscle(s) responsible for these movements (eccentric, concentric, isometric)?

*FORCE COUPLE

21. Connect a 12-ft length of rope to each of the diagonally opposite legs of a table (Figure 1-1).

a. One person pulls rope X in the direction indicated. Pull hard enough to cause the table to move.

b. Now, a second person *independently* (first person stops pulling) pulls rope Y in the direction indicated with enough force to move the table.

c. Describe the movement of the table when each person pulled independently.

d. Now, both people pull simultaneously in the directions indicated and with enough force to cause the table to move.
e. Describe the motion resulting from the simultaneous pull.

The simultaneous pull resulted in a force couple. In this text, examples of muscles acting as force couples on bones are discussed in Chapters 3, 7, and 10.

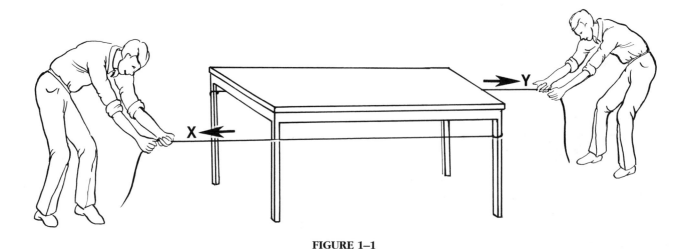

FIGURE 1–1

VECTORS—BASIC PROBLEMS

The remaining problems deal with the graphic illustration of forces, vectors. Additional topics addressed are moment arm, lever systems, torque, resolution of forces, and muscle forces and effects. You will need a metric ruler for this section.

22. Assuming that 1 mm = 1 N (newton), on Figure 1-2 attach a vector representing a force of 12 N to lever AB that will tend to turn the lever clockwise. On the lever diagram, what does the symbol $\wedge$ represent?

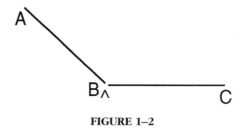

FIGURE 1–2

23. Recall the definition of center of mass from item 16. In lever diagrams, gravity vectors are attached at the assigned center of mass.
   a. All gravity vectors must have what direction?
   b. The length of any gravity vector will depend on what?
   c. The force of gravity on lever CB in Figure 1-2 is 10 N. Which of the following vectors is appropriate to apply as a gravity vector to Figure 1-2?

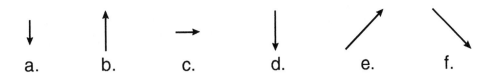

a.   b.   c.   d.   e.   f.

24. Any force applied to a lever can be represented by a vector. The musculoskeletal system can be thought of as a system of levers to which intrinsic and extrinsic forces are applied. Much of the intrinsic force is applied by muscle pull. In the case of muscle forces, the direction of the vector will usually be along the line of pull of the muscle, but the magnitude of the vector is not limited by the distance between the muscle attachments.

   a. Draw a vector representing the muscle force of a muscle whose attachments are x and o in Figure 1–3 below. Note that o is 5 mm from the axis of rotation.

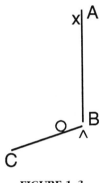

FIGURE 1–3

   b. Why could the vector point in either direction?

   c. How large a force did you draw, given that 1 mm = 1 N?

25. If you have not drawn the muscle force vector to move lever CB in Figure 1–3, fix it now. To find the effectiveness of your muscle force for turning lever CB, you must calculate its torque.

   a. What are the necessary values in the equation defining torque?

   b. Which value is still missing to calculate torque for your muscle force?

   c. Find that value and make the calculation.

   d. Why could you *not* use the given muscle force and the distance from its attachment to the axis as the values to calculate the torque of the muscle?

26. On Figure 1–4, attach a vector to each of the three points of application for the following forces:

   a. The force of gravity on the hand
   b. The force of gravity on the mass of the forearm
   c. A vertical force attached to the forearm that promotes clockwise rotation of the forearm

NOTE: Do not worry about the magnitude of the vectors at this time. Concentrate on the points of attachment and the direction of each.

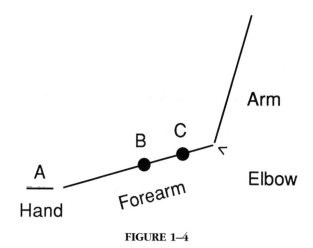

FIGURE 1–4

27. Measure and record, in millimeters, the length of each moment arm in Figure 1–4 of item 26. Consider the axis of rotation to be in the elbow.

    a. _____

    b. _____

    c. _____

28. On Figure 1-5, attach the vector at B that will place the lever system in static equilibrium. Draw the vector to scale.

    AB = 10 mm   AC = 30 mm
    F   = ?   W = 10 N

    a. What class lever is drawn here?
    b. State the basic characteristics of vectors.

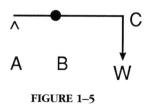

FIGURE 1–5

29. In Figure 1-6, how far from the axis should W_b be placed for the system to be in equilibrium?

    AB = 30 mm   F = 58 N
    AC = 60 mm W_a = 9 N
    AD = ? W_b = 10 N

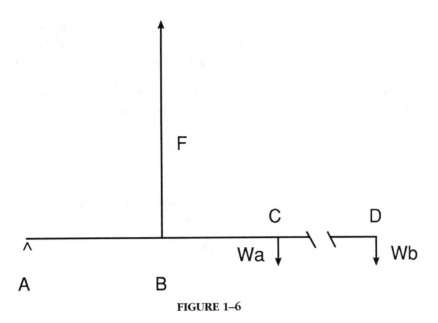

FIGURE 1–6

30. On Figure 1-7, apply a force of the same magnitude as the force in item 24 to the indicated point of attachment on lever CB. Draw it so that it is most effective in producing counterclockwise rotation of the lever CB.

   a. The distance from the attachment of this force to the axis is 5 mm, as it was in item 24, but in this case this distance is the moment arm in the torque calculation. Why?

   b. Compare the torque found in this drawing with the torque calculated in item 26.

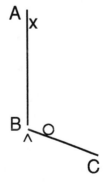

FIGURE 1–7

31. Now, apply a second vector to Figure 1-7 at the same point of attachment and same magnitude as the vector in item 30 that will most effectively compress lever CB onto the point of rotation. The two forces you have drawn should be at a right angle to one another. Their efforts, if applied simultaneously to the lever, can be represented by a single force applied to the same spot.

   a. What defines the magnitude and direction of that single force?

   b. Draw it.

32. On the lever system in Figure 1-8, apply a gravity force of 15 N to the center of mass ($\otimes$) and label it $\mathbf{F_g}$.

   a. The gravity force $\mathbf{F_g}$ has at least two potential effects on the lever, turning it at the point of rotation and separating or compressing (translating) it on lever AB at the point of rotation. Which direction will $\mathbf{F_g}$ tend to turn and translate the lever?

   b. We can find the relative value of the turning and translating forces contained on $\mathbf{F_g}$ by performing the reverse of what we did in item 31. The directions of the turning and translating forces are predetermined. Explain.

   c. At the point of attachment of the original vector, apply the vectors that represent the components of $\mathbf{F_g}$ that are turning (rotary) and compressing or separating (translatory) the levers.

   d. We can be sure the rotary and translatory components you drew for $\mathbf{F_g}$ are proportional by completing the parallelogram for which the original vector is the diagonal. The two components you have drawn are two sides of a rectangle. Draw the other two sides so that they meet at the tip of the original vector at a right angle.

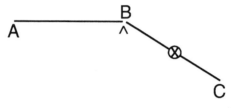

FIGURE 1–8

33. We can apply some of the vector principles to the clinical situation by considering the schematic of a right knee in Figure 1-9. The patient recently had anterior cruciate ligament repair surgery. One function of this ligament is to prevent anterior translation of the tibia on the femur. The therapist has decided to start quadriceps exercise for the patient, resisting the patient with a force of 15 N at the ankle. This force is drawn proportionally on the figure. The distance from the point of application of the resistance force $\mathbf{F_r}$ to the point of rotation is 40 cm. The distance from the point of muscle attachment x to the point of rotation is 7.5 cm. Note that the distances are not drawn to scale.

   a. Draw to scale the rotary component of the effort force of the quadriceps needed to hold this system in static equilibrium, and apply it to the point of attachment of the muscle.

   b. Note that you now have a force couple within the tibia that resembles the one we experimented with in item 21. Where is the center of rotation for this force couple?

   c. What will be the direction of potential rotation for this force couple?

   d. What will be the potential effect on the point of attachment of the tibia at the knee? What structure(s) might this affect?

   e. Should the therapist be sure her liability insurance is paid up?

   f. Bonus question. Why does the situation become worse at full extension of the knee? Assume that the resistance is applied by a machine that is not gravity dependent.

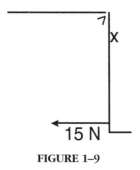

FIGURE 1–9

GLOSSARY OF TERMS

Below is a list of terms that we have found cause difficulty for many students. You will use some of them repeatedly in the course of this chapter, and some are terms regularly used (and misused) in professional practice. Your kinesiology textbook contains most of the definitions. We suggest that you look up the definitions of all the terms now or as you encounter them in the course of dealing with problems in the workbook. Once the definitions are obtained, this glossary will be your ready reference, and will help you with the workbook.

Center of gravity (center of mass):

Force:

Lever:

Lever arm:

Line of gravity:

Moment arm:

Resolution of vectors:

Rotary component force:

Torque:

Translatory component force:

Vector:

ANSWERS TO BIOMECHANICS

NOTE: There may be more than one legitimate answer to several of the problems. The following are the answers considered as first choice by the authors.

1. a. Flexion
   b. Pronation
   c. Supination
   d. Lateral rotation
   e. Medial rotation
   f. Extension
   g. Abduction
   h. Adduction

2. **Ankle**

   Dorsiflexion (flexion)
   Plantarflexion (extension)

   Spine

   Flexion (forward bending)
   Extension (backward bending)
   Lateral flexion (lateral bending)

   Wrist

   Radial deviation (abduction)
   Ulnar deviation (adduction)

3. a. Flexion
   b. Extension
   c. Supination
   d. Pronation

4. a. Extension
   b. Adduction
   c. Flexion

5. Your list should look like this: (Motion) of the (bone) at the (joint). For instance, flexion of the humerus at the shoulder, or extension of the tibia at the knee.

6. a. Flexion of the humerus at the shoulder, extension of the forearm at the elbow
   b. Flexion of the femur at the hip and flexion of the tibia at the knee

*7. Frontal

*8. Transverse

9. The paper is a concrete representation of the imaginary two-dimensional plane.

10. a. The pencil should be in a side-to-side direction
    b. The pencil should be in a front-to-back direction
    c. The pencil should be in an up-and-down direction

11. a. Sagittal and medial-lateral
    b. Frontal and anterior-posterior
    c. Horizontal and vertical

12. a. Sagittal
    b. Frontal

c. Frontal
Transverse
d. Transverse
e. Sagittal
f. Frontal

* 13. This demonstrates the need for the line of gravity to fall within the base of support if the upright position is to be maintained. The smaller the base of support, the more difficult it is to achieve balance, since the line of gravity has such a small area in which it must fall.

* 14. There are many possibilities; one would be to stand on one foot.

* 15. Your body shifts toward the supporting limbs.

* 16. a. Find the balance point, which is the composite center of mass. The same could be done with the class-mate, but only the point along the subject's length could be found this way. Other means are needed to find the intersecting point between the anterior and posterior surfaces of the body.
  b. The center of mass is where the effect of gravity is concentrated in the object.

* 17. a. This is an extension of item 13. The students can either experiment to find the center of mass on one an-other (perhaps using a teeter-totter), or simply use one of their text references to determine its location. Note that the line from the sticker falls within the length of the feet.
  b. This is a demonstration of the shift of the center of mass from the standing to the sitting position. Note that the line from the sticker falls outside the area of the feet.
  c and d. These activities demonstrate the need for the anterior shift of body weight so that the line of grav-ity falls within the base of support prior to attempting to come to a standing position. Note that, as the subject successfully moves from sitting to standing, the center of mass is shifting again, so the stickers are no longer accurate. They do, however, provide a general sense of the interaction of the center of mass and the base of support. This is a basic principle used daily in the practice of motor training or re-training.

* 18. For each of the activities, gravity is the primary force causing the motion.
  a. Elbow flexors are most active, eccentrically.
  b. Trunk and hip extensors are most active, eccentrically.
  c. Knee extensors are most active, eccentrically.

19. Since gravity pulls down, it pulls the body or body part in each example in item 18 and causes the motion de-scribed. The muscles responsible for the opposite motion are active to counteract the effects of gravity.

20. Descriptions:
  a. For 18a, extend the forearm at the elbow, but position the limb so that the hand is rising against gravity, for example, supine with the humerus vertical and starting with the elbow flexed. For 18b, do a sit-up. For 18c, lie prone and flex the tibia at the knee.
  b. The above are suggested solutions that include the positions.
  c. Concentric.

* 21. d. With an independent pull, the table slides in the direction of the force, as well as rotating slightly around a pivot point of one of the legs. This is a combination of translatory (linear) and rotary motion, with most being translatory.
  e. With simultaneous pulling, the table rotates *only*, with the point of rotation being between the points of application of the two forces. This is the definition of the movement produced by a force couple, and a demonstration of a force couple in action.

22. The vector must be attached on the right side of the lever and point to the right. The symbol $\wedge$ represents the point of rotation of the lever diagram.

23. a. All gravity vectors point straight down.

b. Since the vector represents magnitude by how long it is, the gravity vector represents the force applied by the mass of the lever.

c. The correct vector is "d." The vector must be attached to the lever at the symbol for center of mass, be 10 mm long, and point straight down.

24. a. The vector must attach to one of the levers and align between x and o in Figure 1–3.

b. Since a muscle pulls only to the middle, the effect will be determined by which attachment is stable and which is movable. The arrow would generally be in the direction of movement of the mobile lever.

c. Measure the force with your metric ruler.

25. a. The necessary values needed to calculate the torque of a force are the value of the force and the perpendicular distance from the line of the force to the axis of motion (the moment arm).

b. The missing value from the information in Figure 1–3 is the moment arm.

c. You must draw a line that is perpendicular to the muscle force vector but also passes through the axis of motion and measure that line. That value multiplied by the value of your force vector is the torque of that force.

d. You could not use the two obvious values because the line along the lever from the muscle force to the axis is not perpendicular to the line of the muscle force; therefore, it does not fit the definition of moment arm.

26. See Figure 1–10.

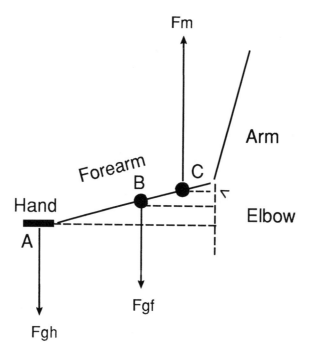

FIGURE 1–10

27. a. 48 mm
   b. 20 mm
   c. 7 mm

28. F = 30 N

a. The lever is a third-class lever with the effort placed between the resistance and the fulcrum.

b. The basic characteristics of a vector are that it has direction, magnitude, and point of application.

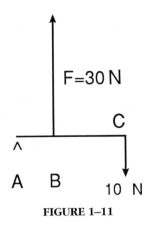

FIGURE 1–11

29. $(AC \times \mathbf{W_a}) + (AD \times \mathbf{W_b}) = AB \times F$

$$AD = \frac{(AB \times F) - (AC \times \mathbf{W_a})}{\mathbf{W_b}}$$

$$AD = \frac{(30 \times 58) - (60 \times 9)}{10}$$

$AD = 120$ mm

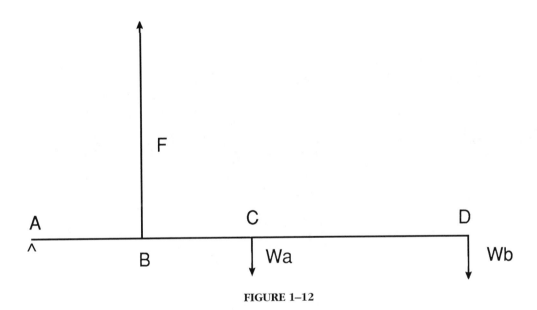

FIGURE 1–12

30. For the force to be *most* effective in turning the lever, it must be applied perpendicular to the lever; otherwise, some of its effort is dissipated in translatory activity, i.e., dragging the lever toward or away from the point of rotation.

    a. Now the distance from the point of attachment of the force to the point of rotation can be used as the moment arm distance because the force is perpendicular to the lever and the distance conforms to the definition of moment arm.

b. The torque calculated for this item will be larger than the one for item 26, since the moment arm is larger.

31. The magnitude and direction of the single force will be determined by the magnitude and direction of the original two forces. We can draw the single force using the parallelogram method. Using dotted lines, finish the parallelogram started by the two vectors you drew. Note that since the two vectors are the same size, the finished parallelogram will be a square. Now draw a vector from the original point of attachment of your first two vectors to the diagonally opposite corner. Put an arrow tip on it, and it is the single vector with the direction and magnitude to accomplish the same effect as the two separate ones. See Figure 1–13 below for an example.

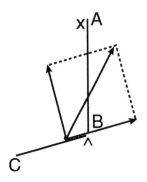

FIGURE 1–13

32. a. Clockwise and separate.
    b. The directions of the most effective turning and translating vectors are predetermined because they have fixed relationships to the lever. The most effective angle for the turning vector is 90° to the lever. The translating force is most effective if it is parallel to the lever. In this case, it points away from the point of rotation, thus separating the levers. The magnitude of these proportional forces will be determined by the original force.
    c and d. See Figure 1–14 below.

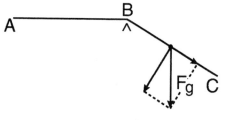

FIGURE 1–14

33. a. See Figure 1-15. To hold the system in static equilibrium, the muscle force must generate 600 N·cm of rotary force (torque). The moment arm available to the muscle is 7.5 cm (since we are using the rotary component of the muscle force). The rotary force of the muscle needed to balance the 15 N resistance is 80 N.
    b. The center of rotation is midway between the two points of application of the forces.
    c. Clockwise.
    d. Anterior translation, stressing the repaired anterior cruciate ligament.
    e. You bet.

f. Because you add the mass of the leg to the resistance being applied to the leg, it must now be opposed by an increase in muscle force. The closer to full extension, the greater the moment arm of the effect of gravity on the mass of the leg. At 90° of flexion, the moment arm of gravity on the mass of the leg is virtually 0. As extension increases, the moment arm also increases, reaching a maximum at 0° of extension.

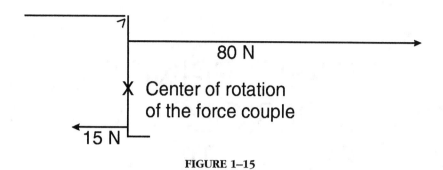

FIGURE 1–15

2 BASIC PRINCIPLES OF KINESIOLOGY AND EVALUATION

ARTHROLOGY

1. In your own words, describe the three major types of joints:
   a. Fibrous joint:

   b. Cartilaginous joint:

   c. Synovial joint:

2. Of the synovial joints, which type(s) has(have):
   a. Three degrees of freedom:

   b. Two degrees of freedom:

   c. One degree of freedom:

*3. Using heavy paper or cardboard, cut out representations, in profile, of the bone ends and part of the long bone shaft of an interphalangeal joint of your index finger. Now:
   a. Actively flex and extend the middle phalanx of your index finger on the proximal phalanx (the middle phalanx moves; the proximal one does not).
   b. Reproduce the movement with the cardboard cutout.
   c. Actively flex and extend the proximal phalanx of your index finger on the middle phalanx (the proximal moves while you hold the middle one still).
   d. Reproduce the movement with the cardboard cutout.

4. Below are drawings of a joint (Figures 2-1 and 2-2). On Figure 2-1, place arrows that will indicate the direction of movement of the convex joint surface and its shaft as it flexes on the stationary concave surface (one arrow for the joint surface and one arrow for the shaft). Label those arrows flexion. Next, on the same drawing, draw a second set of arrows for the convex surface and its shaft as it extends, and label them extension.

 Place arrows on Figure 2-2 indicating flexion and extension of the concave surface as it moves on a stationary convex surface. Place a second set of arrows for flexion and extension of the shaft.

 Your arrows and item 3 demonstrate a principle of movement of convex-concave joint surfaces in relation to the bones to which they are attached.

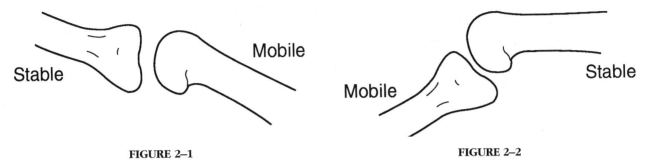

FIGURE 2–1   FIGURE 2–2

a. What is the relationship between the movement of the joint surface and movement of the shaft when a convex surface moves over a concave surface?

b. What is the relationship between the movement of the joint surface and the shaft when a concave surface moves over a convex surface?

c. Now put this in your own words as a principle of motion.

*5. Place a femur at a 30° angle to the surface of a table with both condyles in contact with the surface. The femur should be oriented with the femoral head angled up, rather than down (see Figure 2–3).

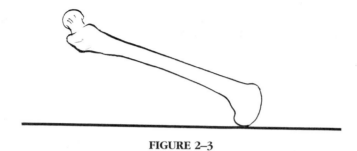

FIGURE 2–3

Now, keep the condyles in contact with the same spot on the table and raise the shaft to vertical.

a. Describe the movement of the femoral condyles at the point of contact with the table as the shaft is moved to vertical.

b. Try the activity again, keeping the condyles in contact with the tabletop, but allowing them to move off the spot as the femur comes to vertical. Describe what you saw occur this time.

*6. Select a partner and have him lie supine on a plinth. You are about to perform joint accessory motions and may need faculty input for confirmation of your technique.

a. You will be examining the left shoulder, so you will be on the left side of the subject with your left hand placed firmly over the anterior aspect of the clavicle to hold the shoulder girdle down on the plinth. Place your right hand beneath the humerus close to the axilla. Grasp the humerus firmly (do not dig your fingers in), press down with your left hand, and pick up with your right hand. Attempt to move the humerus as a unit, keeping it horizontally oriented as it moves. You should see the humerus come up slightly and a slight bulge appear on the anterior shoulder just beneath the acromion.

b. You have just produced an anterior glide mobilization of the glenohumeral joint. Anterior and posterior gliding are accessory movements available in the glenohumeral joint. Inferior glide and lateral distraction are also available in this joint. How could you produce these in your subjects? Try it.

c. What accessory movements can you produce in the metacarpophalangeal (MCP) joint of the index finger of the hand?

Not all accessory movements are passively performed by one individual on another. Some are produced during normal everyday activities. For example, grasp a drink can tightly and watch your fingers closely. You will see them rotating on their long axes to accommodate the pressure. Axial rotation in the fingers is not a movement normally under voluntary control.

*7. Give a definition of accessory joint movement and speculate on its kinesiological usefulness.

*8. a. While relaxed and sitting, put your knee in a position that makes it difficult to move your patella with your fingers; that is, the patella appears to be firmly fixed in that position. What is that position of the knee?

   b. Now put your knee in a position in which it is easy to move your patella. What is that position?

   c. What structures caused the difference in the ease of movement of the patella?

   You have just demonstrated the difference in loose-packed and close-packed positions of the patellofemoral joint.
   d. Passively abduct and adduct the index MCP joint in various positions of flexion and extension. Determine the open- and close-packed positions of that joint.
   e. In your own words, define open-packed position and close-packed position.
   Open-packed:

   Close-packed:

*9. Standing erect, flex your right humerus at the shoulder, keeping your elbow extended so that your hand is out in front of you. Now:
   a. Bend and straighten your right elbow.
   b. Grasp an immovable object and bend your right elbow (you will have to move your body in order to allow your elbow to bend).
   c. Which situation was the open kinematic chain and which was the closed chain?

d. How many and which joints moved in a and how many in b?

10. There are no muscles that control elbow movement *and* have a line of pull that crosses the medial or lateral aspect of the joint. Why?

*11. a. Observe a partner and determine the number of cardinal planes in which each of the following joints can voluntarily move.
   - MCP joint of the index finger
   - PIP (proximal interphalangeal) joint of the index finger
   - Knee joint
   - Humeroulnar joint
   - Hip joint
   The joints that allow movement in one plane have one degree of freedom; in two planes, two degrees, and so on.
   b. Now observe which of the joints can perform circumduction and associate that observation with the degrees of freedom available to that joint.

MYOLOGY

*12. For this activity, you will need a piece of string at least 2 ft long or a rubber band and an articulated skeleton. Place the string or rubber band across the appropriate joint so that if it were a shortening muscle pulling one attachment toward the other, the following motions would occur:
   a. Abduction of the femur at the hip
   b. Extension of the hand at the wrist
   c. Adduction of the humerus at the shoulder
   d. Flexion with supination of the forearm at the elbow
   e. Extension of the femur at the hip with flexion of the tibia at the knee

13. The string in item 12 represents the line of pull of the muscle involved. For each muscle represented in item 12, describe the orientation and direction of the muscle's line of pull to the axis of joint motion. Orientation means anterior or posterior, medial or lateral, superior or inferior. Direction of the line of pull could be in an anterior-to-posterior direction, medial-to-lateral direction, inferior-to-superior direction, or their opposites.
   a.
   b.
   c.
   d.
   e.

*14. You will need a cut rubber band or straight piece of elastic for this activity. Select a partner and place one end of the rubber band on the proximal sternum. *Slightly* stretch the band and hold the other end in place on the subject's *right* mastoid process. Ask the subject to move his head in the direction of the line of pull of the rubber band as you allow it to contract.
   You should see the combined movement of turning the head toward the left and tipping toward the right and forward as the rubber band shortens.
   NOTE: Be sure to move the head to a point that brings the rubber band to its shortest length. That point best demonstrates the combined action of unilateral sternocleidomastoid action.

You have just demonstrated the action of a unilateral pull of the sternocleidomastoid muscle. Now describe the relationship and direction of the line of pull of the muscle to the axis of motion for each of the component motions described.

a. Rotation of the head on the neck

b. Lateral bending of the head and neck

c. Flexion of the upper cervical spine on the lower cervical spine

*15. From a position of sitting on the floor with your legs straight in front of you, perform an eccentric contraction of your iliopsoas muscles bilaterally. In what position are you now?

*16. From this new position, perform a concentric contraction of your neck flexors and maintain this new position for a slow count of 20. Describe the position you were holding. What type of contraction were your neck muscles performing *while you were counting* to 20?

*17. a. Name the prime mover for extension of the femur at the hip.
  b. Is it the agonist or antagonist for that movement?
  c. Is it the agonist or antagonist for flexion of the femur at the hip?
  d. Name a synergist for extending the femur at the hip.
  e. Slowly move from a standing position to sitting in a chair and feel the contraction in the prime mover for hip extension. What function did the contraction in the prime mover play during the move from standing to sitting?

  f. From a standing position, slowly step up onto a surface at least 12 inches high and feel the contraction in the prime mover for hip extension. What function did the contraction in the prime mover play during stepping up?

  g. What type of muscle contraction (eccentric, concentric, isometric) was performed in e and f?

18. Since the prime mover for extension of the femur at the hip can also produce lateral rotation of the femur, some other muscle(s) must be active when you perform extension of the femur at the hip without simultaneous lateral rotation. A muscle performing this function is called a neutralizing synergist or neutralizer. What muscles(s) about the hip could serve this function for the prime mover, thus allowing pure extension?

REVERSE ACTIONS

*19. Perform the following movements:
  a. Flex your hip, but keep your femur stable.
  b. Dorsiflex your ankle, but keep your foot flat on the floor.
  c. Find a way to extend your knee, but keep your tibia stable.
     Name each of these actions according to the Rule of Three. All of these are reverse actions.

* 20. Reverse actions can also be accomplished with eccentric contractions.

    a. Demonstrate the reverse action of the pelvis moving on the femur with the primary force provided by gravity and controlled by an eccentric contraction.

    b. Based on items 19 and 20, develop a definition of the concept of reverse action.

GONIOMETRY BASICS

* 21. Use a blackboard or a large piece of paper and place two dots on it that determine a line. Place the stationary arm of a goniometer on the surface so that the dots fall on the centerline of the goniometer. Now, place two more dots on the surface to describe a line that is close to and will intersect with the first line (these two lines should form one angle, not an X). Keeping the first two dots under the midline of the stationary arm, align the movable arm of the goniometer so that the second set of dots falls on the centerline of that arm. (Depending on where you placed the second two dots, you may have to slide the goniometer up or down to get the movable arm over the second two dots.) Read the angle on the goniometer.

* 22. Repeat exercise 21, but this time place all four dots on the surface before you align the goniometer. Be sure that the two lines described by the four dots intersect at some point (to form one angle, not an X). Align the goniometer arms so that they form the angle described by the two lines. Read the angle. Take the goniometer off and close it. Have a second person repeat the measurement and compare measurements.

* 23. You will need a Ping-Pong ball to complete the next task. If you are using a blackboard, you will hang the ball from a string. If you are using paper, simply place the ball over an area representing one of the dots.

    Place two dots on the blackboard or paper to describe a line. Place one dot and the Ping-Pong ball for the second dot to represent another line that will intersect with the first. Do not hold the ball in place. Place the goniometer over the ball and its dot, being sure the goniometer is in contact with the ball as you take the measurement. Measure the angle described by the two lines. Take the goniometer off and close it. Have a second person repeat the measurement. Compare the results of item 22 and this activity for:

    a. Ease of obtaining an accurate measurement

    b. Reproducibility of results

24. Assuming that we can study the body as a system of levers and axes, state whatever principles of goniometric measurement you understand as a result of items 21 to 23. In your deliberation, consider:

    a. The definition of a line

    b. The importance of stability of each reference landmark (point)

    c. The relative importance of the placement of the axis of the goniometer versus the placement of the arms of the goniometer during measurement

    Principles:

* 25. a. With a small group of students (3 to 5), generate reasonable landmarks for measuring abduction of the humerus at the shoulder, internal rotation of the femur on the pelvis, and extension of the humerus at the shoulder. Do *not* consult your goniometry text for this activity.

    b. After you identify the landmarks, generate as many ways as you can of substituting other motions for abduction of the humerus at the shoulder with the person standing, internal rotation of the femur on the pelvis with the person sitting on a treatment table, and extension of the humerus at the shoulder with the person standing.

c. Now determine how you could avoid those substitutions that you just identified.

d. Have at least two people measure each motion using the landmarks that you identified.

e. Identify any additional principles of goniometry that you have discovered and add them to the list you made in item 24.

MANUAL MUSCLE-TESTING BASICS

*26. Have your subject sit on the edge of the treatment table with his feet dangling. Have him flex the right forearm at the elbow to about 120°. Grasp the wrist of the flexed arm with your right hand and ask the subject to keep the elbow flexed and his left hand behind his back. (Note: This is a modification of the muscle-testing position for biceps. Consult a muscle-testing text for an illustration.) Instruct him not to lean back and not to support himself with the left hand. Now, gradually pull on the right wrist in an attempt to straighten the elbow. Pull until you obtain a reaction from the subject. What reaction did you obtain?

Now, place your left hand in front of the subject's right shoulder, your palm to his shoulder, and push against the shoulder as you pull with your right hand. Pull hard with your right hand, but do not allow the shoulder to come forward.

a. In which exercise did the subject resist more strongly with elbow flexion?

b. In the second part of this activity, you stabilized your partner. Now state a use or uses of stabilization in the performance of manual muscle testing.

*27. Select two subjects, each with the shoulders exposed. One subject should have a large frame and well-defined shoulder girdle musculature. The other should be slightly built with relatively small shoulder girdle musculature. Seat the subjects on low stools. Stand behind the larger subject and ask him to abduct the humerus at the shoulder to 90° bilaterally. Place your hand just above the elbow and have the subject resist while you push down vigorously. How much resistance can you apply? Can you break the contraction? Now, resist the slightly built subject in the same way. Could you break that contraction? Answer the following questions:

a. Is either subject considered abnormal?

b. Were you able to apply maximal resistance to each subject?

c. Define maximal resistance.

* 28. a. On the slightly built subject, with the humerus abducted 90° at the shoulder, apply your downward force just above the elbow, but at an acute angle rather than perpendicular to the humerus; have most of your force directed laterally rather than downward. Compare the force you needed to apply in this exercise with the force you used in item 27. Was there a difference in the amount of force you had to apply to break the contraction? Why?

   b. With the same subject, repeat the process but place your resisting hand on the humerus just distal to the shoulder joint rather than close to the elbow. Apply your resistance perpendicular to the humerus. Compare the force you exerted to break the abduction contraction this time to the force you used in item 27 and in a, above. Relate your findings in items 27 and 28a and b to the principles of resistance application outlined in your muscle-testing text.

* 29. Select a subject who has well-developed shoulder musculature and normal shoulder structure. Ask the subject to assume the position described in item 27. Tell the subject that you will be applying maximum pressure and ask the subject to fix the shoulders as well as he can. Place your hands at the elbows and apply downward pressure firmly and *quickly*. You will see the arms go down slightly, even though the subject is strong and was theoretically prepared for the resistance. Repeat the procedure and build your resistance slowly. The arms will not go down.

   How do these findings relate to the technique of applying resistance in a manual muscle-testing break test?

* 30. Select a subject who is dressed in loose-fitting shorts. Place this subject so that he performs an active extension of the femur at the hip from the anatomical position or 0° starting position. The movement must be accomplished without gravity resisting or assisting the movement and with the limb supported on a plinth. (Hint: You may have to assist the subject for balance.) Perform the same activity for abduction of the humerus at the shoulder, flexion of the forearm at the elbow, and flexion of the tibia at the knee. In each case, have the subject complete a full range of motion. How did you decide that gravity was not resisting or assisting the motions? In what plane did each of the motions take place?

  31. With one or two classmates, discuss whether or not manual muscle testing (MMT) would be useful in assessing muscle strength for the following problems:

   a. Lack of function due to a long period in bed

   b. Lack of function due to pain during motion

   c. Lack of function due to a brain injury

  d. Lack of function because of pressure on a nerve

  e. Lack of function due to lack of motion

PALPATION BASICS

The following exercises are designed to allow you structured feedback about the effects of your touch/palpation on a subject and to help you learn some of the basic principles of successful palpation. For these activities to achieve their ends, the subject must tell the person doing the palpation what he feels (comfort or discomfort, safe or unsafe, etc.). It is much better to obtain that information from a student colleague than from a patient in the clinic.

* 32. As therapist, communicate through touch the following attitudes to your subject. Do not use words and perform the activities in random order. The subject is to tell the therapist what the attitude is that is being conveyed. During the activities, the therapist should compare how relaxed the subject felt under each of the circumstances.

    The therapist tries to impart a sense of:

  a. Confidence and competence while performing passive flexion of the head on the neck (subject supine with head off the end of the plinth)
  b. Tentativeness and apprehension during passive flexion of the head on the neck (subject in same position)
  c. Care and concern, attending to the patient during passive knee flexion and extension
  d. Being rushed and impersonal during passive knee flexion and extension

* 33. Palpate, and then analyze what you had to do in order to sucessfully palpate, each of the following items. Remember, the subject should continue to provide feedback to the therapist concerning the nonverbal cues delivered and the comfort of the palpation.

  a. Radial pulse
  b. Acromion
  c. Radial head
  d. Sternocleidomastoid (SCM) muscle from origin to insertion
  Analysis:

* 34. Palpate a contraction in the pronator teres muscle as differentiated from the wrist and finger flexors. What did you have to do in order to confirm that you were palpating the pronator teres, and to differentiate the pronator teres from the flexors?

GLOSSARY OF TERMS

Following is a list of terms that we have found cause difficulty for many students. You will use some of them repeatedly in the course of this chapter, and some are terms regularly used (and misused) in professional practice. Your kinesiology textbook contains most of the definitions. We suggest that you look up the definitions of all the terms now or as you encounter them in the course of dealing with problems in the workbook. Once the definitions are obtained, this glossary will be your ready reference, and will help you with the workbook.

Active insufficiency/passive insufficiency (two terms):

Agonist:

Antagonist:

Close-packed/open-packed positions (two terms):

Concentric:

Contraction:

Contracture:

Eccentric:

Isokinetic:

Isometric:

Isotonic:

Length-tension relationship:

Open kinematic chain/closed kinematic chain (two terms):

Reverse action:

Synergist:

ANSWERS TO BASIC PRINCIPLES OF KINESIOLOGY AND EVALUATION

NOTE: There may be more than one legitimate answer to several of the problems. The following are the answers considered first choices by the authors.

1. Since it is to be written in your own words, a preferred answer is incongruous. Major concepts that should be addressed include the following:

    Fibrous joint: minimal motion; tough, fibrous tissue joining bones
    Cartilaginous joint: limited motion; cartilaginous tissue joining bones
    Synovial joint: freely moving; joint surrounded by fibrous capsule that is lined with synovial membrane

2. a. Ball and socket (triaxial)
    b. Condyloid and saddle or sellar (biaxial)
    c. Hinge or ginglymus and pivot (uniaxial)

*3. This activity gives a concrete demonstration of the convex-concave rule. The information as to which surface is convex and which is concave will be needed prior to attempting the activity. Next, the movement of the "joint surfaces" of the paper cutouts must be observed closely to learn the direction of slide of the joint surface in relation to the direction of movement of the bone.

4. a. The movements occur in opposite directions.
    b. Movement occurs in the same direction.
    c. Your wording of the principle should have the information in a and b, above, combined with the types of joint surfaces involved.

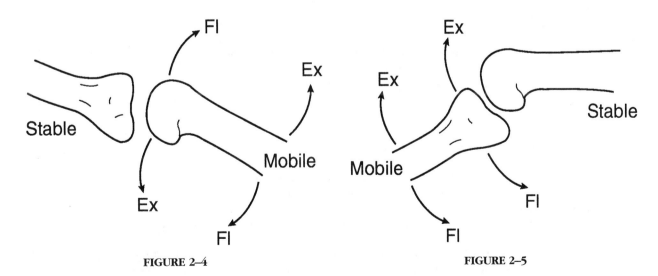

FIGURE 2–4   FIGURE 2–5

*5. a. Demonstrates the need for slide (glide) for the femur to flex and extend on the tibia and maintain its position on the tibial plateau.
    b. Demonstrates the effect of rolling of the femoral condyles without simultaneous glide.

*6. a. Self-explanatory.
  b. For inferior glide, gently but firmly pull the humerus down along the subject's side while stabilizing the scapula. For lateral distraction, stabilize the scapula and gently but firmly pull the proximal humerus directly away from the scapula. The humeral shaft must stay parallel to the trunk for each of these motions.
  c. Anterior-posterior glide, medial-lateral glide, rotation, distraction. To see these, stabilize the metacarpal and firmly grasp the first phalanx of the index finger. Gently move the phalanx so that the proximal end performs the above movements.

7. Joint accessory movement is movement not under volitional control. It allows for conformation of body parts around objects (as in the grip of the hand); deformation of the joint under stress, thus reducing the chance of injury; and greater range of motion than would be otherwise allowed. Other possibilities for answers undoubtedly exist.

*8. a and b. As the knee becomes more flexed, it becomes more difficult to passively move the patella, especially after 30° of knee flexion.
  c. The medial and lateral lips of the patellar articulating surface, the vertical ridge on the posterior surface of the patella, the tightening patellar retinaculum, and the tightening patellar ligament all aid in stabilizing the patella.
  d. The close-packed position of the index MCP (metacarpophalangeal) joint is about 70° of flexion. This can be seen by the decreased mobility of the joint in that position.
  e. Include statements about tension in the ligaments, congruity between bony surfaces, and mobility and stability of the joint.

*9. c. The open kinematic chain is a, and the closed chain is b.
  d. Only one joint moved (the elbow) in a, whereas in b movement at one joint affects the position *of all of the* other joints in the chain so that three joints moved (wrist, elbow, and shoulder).

*10. The structure of the bones and ligaments making up the joint limit the movements to one plane, thus eliminating the necessity for muscles to control movements in the other planes.

11. a. MCP: two planes
    PIP: one plane
    Tibiofemoral: two planes
    Humeroulnar: one plane
    Hip: three planes

  b. Joints with two or three degrees of freedom can perform circumduction.

*12. The emphasis of this activity is to note the orientation of the string to the joint and the direction of the line of the string, once the effective position has been decided. This information can then be correlated with the anatomical information available for the muscles that produce the motion. This activity reinforces the need to learn the location of the attachments of a muscle in order to determine the muscle's probable action.

13. a. Lateral to the hip, running in a superior-inferior direction
  b. Posterior (dorsal) to the wrist, running in a proximal-distal direction
  c. Medial and inferior to the shoulder, running in a medial-lateral direction
  d. Anterior to the elbow and medial to the radius, running in a superior-inferior direction, wrapping medially around the radius
  e. Posterior to the hip and also to the knee, running in a superior-inferior direction

*14. This activity is an effective means of learning about combined actions of a muscle, generally, and the unilateral action of the sternocleidomastoid muscle, specifically.

  a. Anterior to the axis for rotation, running in a superior-lateral to inferior-medial direction
  b. Lateral to the axis for lateral bending, running in a superior to inferior direction
  c. Anterior to the axis for cervical flexion and extension, running in a superior to inferior direction

*15. Supine. Demonstrates the definition of eccentric contraction.

*16. Supine with neck flexed. Demonstrates the definitions of concentric and isometric contractions.

*17. a. Gluteus maximus
   b. Agonist
   c. Antagonist
   d. Hamstring group
   e. Slowed or controlled descent
   f. Elevated the body weight against gravity
   g. (e) Lengthening or eccentric, (f) shortening or concentric

18. You must search for a prime medial rotator of the hip since it can act as antagonist to the lateral rotation component of the gluteus maximus action. The most likely candidate is the gluteus minimus.

*19. For now, it is important to describe the motion using the Rule of Three, because it is much more exact and aids in diminishing confusion while you are still developing the concept of reverse action. Naming the motions by the Rule of Three is as follows:
   a. Flexion of the pelvis at the hip
   b. Dorsiflexion of the tibia at the ankle
   c. Extension of the femur at the knee
       The problems lend themselves to multiple appropriate solutions, so this activity needs faculty input for confirmation of the various solutions.

*20. a. Again, the problems allow for many solutions and require faculty feedback. One example could be standing and bending forward or backward at the waist. The pelvis is moving on the femur while gravity is providing the force producing the movement. The function of the muscles is to control the movement by slowly elongating.
   b. Reverse action is movement of a proximal (usually stationary) segment on the stationary distal (usually moving) one. Reverse actions most often occur in a situation with the distal segment fixed as in a closed kinematic chain.

*21. This activity begins the manipulation of the goniometer and the process of emphasizing the importance of identifying bony landmarks that describe the lines used to perform goniometric measurement.

*22. This activity emphasizes the reproducibility of findings as well as reinforcing the use of landmarks. The angle was found without the need to place the axis of the goniometer in a specific location. This is true for performing clinical goniometry as well. The reasons are based in geometry; the angle formed by lines superimposed over or parallel to the lines of an angle describe the same angle. Therefore, locating the mechanical axis of the body with the axis of the goniometer is superfluous and needlessly time consuming.

*23. This activity works well to demonstrate that the landmarks must be stable in order to obtain accurate and reproducible results.

24. A line is defined by the connection of two points. The two points used to describe the line for goniometry are best if they are observable, stationary, and on the same bone. As soon as the reference points for the two lines are aligned under the arms of the goniometer, the angle described represents the joint angle, and the axis placement becomes immaterial.
    A basic assumption used in this text is that the two lines that define the angle also define the axis by the point of intersection of the two lines. Therefore, *placement of the axis of the goniometer is an unnecessary step*.

25. a. Reasonable landmarks would be anything that remains constant within the body. That usually, but not always, means bones. Some possibilities for shoulder abduction might be the sternum, vertebral column, clavicle, head of the humerus, line of the humerus, and lateral epicondyle of the humerus. As you can see, any landmarks on the levers that you are assessing can be used. There are standards that you need to be aware of but that will come later as you study specific goniometry for each joint. Here we are looking at

principles of goniometry, not specific techniques. Since almost any landmarks on the levers that you are assessing that are visible during the motion are reasonable choices, landmarks for the other two motions will not be listed. Check with your instructor to see if your answers are reasonable.

b. Again, the number of ways to substitute are numerous. Common substitutions are:
- Lateral flexion of the spine to the opposite side for abduction of the humerus at the shoulder
- Elevation of the pelvis on the same side for internal rotation of the femur on the pelvis
- Forward bending of the trunk for extension of the humerus at the shoulder.

c. One way of stabilizing is to instruct the patient not to perform substitution. Sometimes that works, but sometimes you need to do more. Measuring the shoulder with the patient supine or prone can limit lateral flexion or forward bending of the spine. Bilateral internal rotation of the hip will eliminate pelvic elevation as a substitution. Other ways of limiting motion are available also. One way is to have a second person stabilize the patient; this is not often feasible in the clinic.

d. How consistent were you with each other's measurements?

e. Points that you might want to add are:
- Stabilization of the parts that you do not want moving (i.e., the trunk during shoulder abduction, the pelvis during hip rotation).
- Communication with the patient is important.
- Sometimes you may choose a landmark that is not on the body (e.g., the use of a line perpendicular to the ground for a reference in hip rotation). When you do that, it is critical to limit the patient's use of substitutions. For instance, in measuring abduction of the femur at the hip, you are using landmarks on the pelvis and the femur. Therefore, if the pelvis moves, you will know it. However, in measuring rotation of the femur at the hip, your landmarks are on the femur and relative to the floor. Therefore, if the pelvis moves, you will not necessarily know it unless you watch for it.
- There may be other principles. Check with your instructor to confirm your answers.

*26. The most likely result is to have the subject fall or tip forward and release the contraction that was maintaining elbow flexion.

a. The subject was able to resist more strongly with the stabilization force applied to the anterior shoulder.

b. Stabilization allows for a better performance by the muscles tested.

*27. a. No, neither subject is likely to be abnormal.

b. Yes, you were able to apply maximal resistance.

c. This exercise demonstrates the principle that maximal resistance is defined by the qualities of the patient, not by the strength of the therapist. Therefore, a maximal contraction for a healthy 26-year-old is different from that of a healthy 3-year-old or 89-year-old, as well as different between men and women (usually) and among subjects with various body types and builds. This provides a level of subjectivity to the skill of manual muscle testing that is overcome to some degree as one experiences many different subjects. One of the purposes of practicing on your classmates is to begin to define the range of "normal" strength.

*28. a. This activity demonstrates the effectiveness of the therapist's resistance applied at various angles. For reproducibility of results across time and across patients, and for maintenance of efficiency of effort, the best angle at which to apply resistance is 90° to the part. Force applied 90° to a lever provides a pure rotary effort, and thus is most effective in attempting to turn the lever on its axis.

b. For the best mechanical advantage and control, the therapist applies resistance at the most distal point on the bony lever. We have found it best not to cross subsequent joints to apply the resistance.

*29. In order to give the patient the best opportunity to demonstrate the available strength of a muscle, the resistance must build slowly to allow recruitment of motor units.

*30. Different solutions are possible for these problems. Each solution will have the motion occur parallel to the ground (perpendicular to the gravity line). Since the plane of motion is in relation to the body, it remains the same, that is, sagittal for hip extension and frontal for shoulder abduction. In each case, the plane of movement is parallel to the ground.

31. a. Lack of function due to a long period in bed—MMT would be useful for assessing muscle function because there has been no impairment of the control of the muscle.

b. Lack of function due to pain during motion—MMT would not be as useful because you would not know if strength were limited from pain or from muscle pathology.

c. Lack of function due to a brain injury—MMT would not be useful because the muscle may not be getting proper commands from the brain and may be unable to function voluntarily. The problem in this instance is with the brain, not the muscle.

d. Lack of function because of pressure on a nerve—MMT would be useful because the pressure on the nerve can cause muscle weakness but will not cause inappropriate commands to be sent to the muscle.

e. Lack of function due to a lack of motion—MMT would be useful if there is motion at the joint. However, the definitions of grades that are related to range of motion may not apply to these circumstances. When a person does not have full range of motion, he may or may not have normal strength. So, when full range of motion is not available, special notation of the strength grades may need to be made.

*32. Self-explanatory. This activity is best followed by a faculty-led discussion.

*33. For each of the items palpated, the therapist needed to know the anatomical location in relation to the surface anatomy. This can be found in a book. Then, to successfully palpate each, the following had to be done:

a. Both the subject and therapist had to hold still to be able to continually palpate the radial pulse.

b. The therapist had to move his fingers around the area to determine the area or dimensions of the acromion while the subject remained still.

c. The therapist placed fingers over the location of the radial head, then rotated the radius while holding the fingers still. This allowed for confirmation that the radial head was being palpated.

d. The therapist also had to know the action of the SCM in order to ask for its contraction. Then the contraction had to be maintained while the length of the muscle was palpated.

The general principles of palpation operating here are: if the object of the palpation moves, the therapist must hold still to feel it as it moves; if the object is stationary, the therapist must move to feel it.

*34. In order to palpate a muscle that is anatomically close to several others, the therapist must ask for the particular action of that muscle, and then ask for a minimal contraction in order to obtain action of only that muscle. In this example, the contraction in the pronator teres will not be felt if the common flexors of the forearm are activated simultaneously. Thus a minimal contraction of the pronator is requested when attempting to palpate only that muscle.

3 SPINE AND PELVIS

OSTEOLOGY OF THE SPINE AND PELVIS

1. Divide the 33 vertebrae into their respective categories and indicate the number of vertebrae in each segment.

2. Label the parts of a vertebra (Figure 3-1), including: body, pedicles, lamina, transverse processes, spinous process, and facet joints.

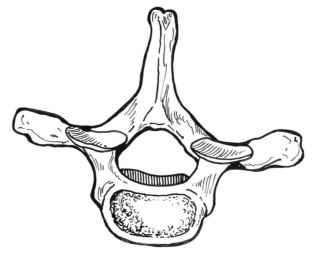

FIGURE 3–1

3. Identify the condyles of the occiput on a skeleton. Are they representative of a convex or concave surface?

*4. Describe (draw and label) the normal curves of the vertebral column from the lateral view. Indicate which are primary and which are secondary curves. Why are the curves named primary and secondary?

5. Name the bones that make up the pelvis.

*6. The functions of the pelvis are to:
   • Connect the vertebral column to the lower limbs
   • Transmit forces from the lower limbs to the vertebral column
   • Support the abdomen

   On a model of a pelvis, identify the following parts or structures:

   Iliac crest   Lesser sciatic notch
   Anterior superior iliac spine   Ischial spine
   Posterior superior iliac spine   Ischial tuberosity
   Greater sciatic notch   Pubic crest

7. Define a spinal segment. Describe the exit of a spinal nerve from its respective spinal segment. Include the structure through which it exits and the relationship of the vertebral level and the spinal cord level in your answer.

8. Identify the boundaries of the intervertebral foramen. Label them on Figure 3-2.

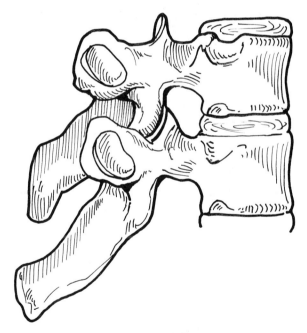

FIGURE 3–2

9. What is the significance of a change in size of the intervertebral foramen?

10. Locate the level at which the spinal cord ends. What is the bundle of nerves below the termination of the spinal cord called?

ARTHROLOGY OF THE SPINE AND PELVIS

11. Identify the types of joints involved in the following articulations:

    Vertebral body-to-vertebral body

    Facet-to-facet

    Pubis-to-pubis

    Sacrum-to-ilium

12. Identify the intrajoint motions available to the joint articulations listed below. Intrajoint motions could be gliding, rotation, or spinning. They are not the resultant classical motions of flexion, extension, and so on.

    Vertebral body-to-vertebral body

    Facet-to-facet

    Pubis-to-pubis

    Sacrum-to-ilium

*13. The following table summarizes the planes and axes of spinal movements.

Movement	Plane	Axis
Flexion/extension	Sagittal	Medial-lateral direction (intersection of transverse and frontal planes)
Lateral flexion	Frontal	Anterior-posterior direction (intersection of sagittal and transverse planes)
Rotation	Transverse	Superior-inferior direction (intersection of sagittal and frontal planes)

   Now, take a stiff piece of paper and a pencil. As you perform each of the motions listed above, place the paper in the plane of the motion and the pencil along the axis of the motion. Note that the motions occur at many joints, so your placement of axes need not be specific, but rather represent the general orientation of the axis.

14. The planes and axes have been drawn on the diagrams below (Figures 3-3 to 3-5). Label both the planes and the axes.

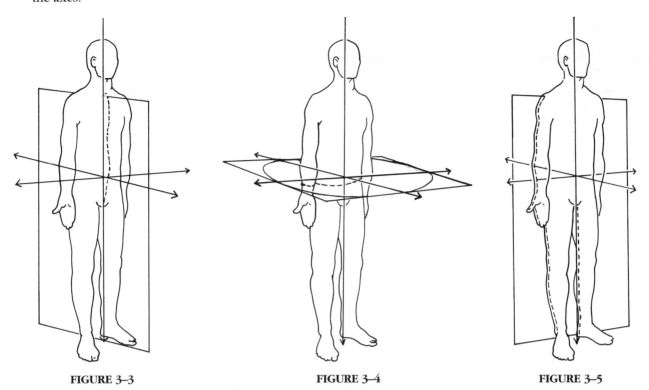

FIGURE 3–3   FIGURE 3–4   FIGURE 3–5

*15. Following is a summary of motions available in the spine. Perform this activity in groups of five, and analyze the motions on all five subjects (more subjects give you a broader idea of what is normal). As you observe your subjects, pick some landmarks to observe. Bony landmarks that are prominent and easily visible are most useful. For instance, the center of the chin can be useful for assessing neck motion; the acromion process can be useful in assessing trunk rotation. In your analysis and on the chart below, note in which portion of the spine most of the motion occurs. In the box representing the spinal section where most of the motion takes place, write a 1; the next most mobile section would be rated 2; and so forth.

	Head (head, C-1, C-2)	Neck (C-3 to C-7)	Thoracic (T-1 to T-12)	Lumbar (L-1 to L-5)
Flexion				
Extension				
Lateral Flexion				
Rotation				

Also note other observations in the chart. Is the motion smooth; is it symmetrical; is there anything that looks unusual?

What motions were easily demonstrated or observed using the landmarks you chose? What motions were difficult to observe using the landmarks you chose?

16. Complete the chart that follows for the ligaments of the vertebral column. The supraspinous ligament has been completed for you as an example.

Ligament	Location
Neck	
Apical	
Alar	
Cruciform	
Tectorial membrane	
Anterior atlanto-occipital	
Posterior atlanto-occipital	
Ligamentum nuchae	
Thoracic and Lumbar	
Supraspinous	Extends from tip of a spinous process to the tip of the spinous process below
Interspinous	
Ligamentum flavum	

Posterior longitudinal

Anterior longitudinal

Intertransverse

Capsular ligaments of the facet

---

17. Identify and label the indicated ligaments of the vertebral column on Figures 3-6 to 3-8.

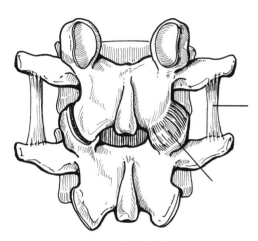

FIGURE 3–6

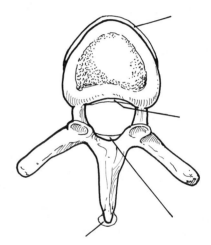

FIGURE 3–7

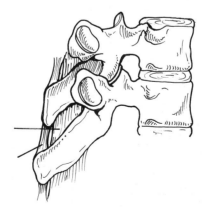

FIGURE 3–8

18. For each of the ligaments listed, indicate which motions it will limit. Refer to Figures 3–6 to 3–8 as you answer this question, although not all ligaments are represented in the diagrams.

    Apical

    Alar

    Cruciform

    Tectorial membrane

    Anterior atlanto-occipital

    Posterior atlanto-occipital

    Ligamentum nuchae

    Supraspinous

    Interspinous

    Ligamentum flavum

    Posterior longitudinal

    Anterior longitudinal

    Intertransverse

Capsular ligaments of the facet joints

19. a. Identify the following ligaments of the pelvis on Figure 3-9:

Iliolumbar ligament
Sacroiliac ligament
Sacrospinous ligament
Sacrotuberous ligament

b. What are the functions of each of the ligaments?

Iliolumbar ligament

Sacroiliac ligament

Sacrospinous ligament

Sacrotuberous ligament

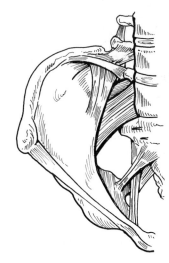

FIGURE 3–9

20. Why does movement at the symphysis pubis always accompany movement of the ilium at the sacroiliac joint?

21. Note the shape of the sacrum as it lies between the ilia (consult your text or Figures 4-3 and 4-4). It can be described as a wedge. You can much more easily induce passive motion in this joint with the subject lying than you can with her sitting or standing. What has sacral shape to do with that fact?

MYOLOGY OF THE SPINE AND PELVIS

Muscles of the Back

The muscles of the back proper are best learned as layers. Their actions can be determined by knowing specific attachments on proximal and distal vertebrae, and knowing whether the muscle is acting unilaterally or bilaterally. The actions can change significantly between unilateral and bilateral action.

Use the following sheets to aid in learning the origin, insertion, and innervation of the muscles of the spine and pelvis. For each muscle named, draw in the muscle on the sketch and fill in the indicated information on the outline.

In all the myology sections, the following abbreviations will be used:

O: Origin of muscle
 I: Insertion of muscle
N: Innervation (both spinal level and peripheral nerve)
R: Relationship of muscle to the axis of motion
A: Action of muscle

Deep Layer of Back Muscles

The deepest layer of back muscles consists of two groups: the intertransversarii and the interspinales.

22. Intertransversarii

    O: Transverse process
    I: Transverse process
    N:
    R: Posterior to axis for flexion and extension; lateral to axis for side bending
    A:

23. Interspinales

    O: Spinous process
    I: Spinous process
    N:
    R:
    A:

Second Layer of Back Muscles

The second layer of muscles can be grouped together and called the transversospinal muscles because of the direction of their fibers in relation to the spinal column. Separately, they are called semispinalis, multifidus, and rotatores. Again, complete the outline below (Figure 3-10), and label the diagram.

24. Semispinalis (spans 3-5 joints)

    O: Transverse process of lower vertebra
    I: Spinous process of higher vertebra
    N:
    R: Wraps around the vertical axis; posterior to axis for flexion and extension
    A: Rotation of the body to opposite side; extension if working bilaterally

25. Multifidus (spans 2-3 joints)

    O: Transverse process of lower vertebra
    I: Spinous process of higher vertebra
    N:
    R:
    A:

26. Rotatores (spans 1-2 joints)

    O:
    I:
    N:
    R:
    A:

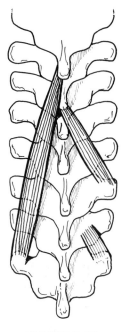

FIGURE 3–10

Third Layer of Back Muscles

The third layer of muscles of the back is the most superficial layer of muscles and can be viewed as three columns. From lateral to medial, they are: cervical, thoracic, and lumbar iliocostalis; longissimus capitis, cervicis, and thoracic; and capitis, cervicis, and thoracic spinales. Note that some additional information has been requested in the outline in relation to unilateral or bilateral action of the muscles.

27. Iliocostalis

    O:

     I:

    N:

    R:

    A: Unilateral contraction:

        Bilateral contraction:

28. Longissimus

    O:

     I:

    N:

    R:

    A: Unilateral contraction:

        Bilateral contraction:

29. Spinales

    O:

     I:

    N:

    R:

    A: Unilateral contraction:

        Bilateral contraction:

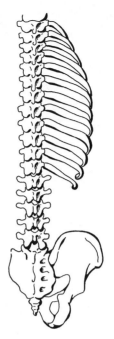

FIGURE 3–11

Anterior Trunk and Abdominal Wall Muscles

30. Psoas major

    O:

     I:

    N:

    R:

    A:

31. Iliacus

    O:

     I:

    N:

    R:

    A:

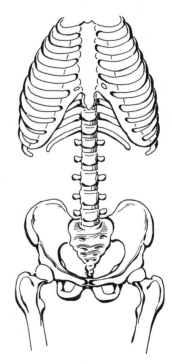

FIGURE 3–12

32. External oblique

    O:

     I:

    N:

    R:

    A: Unilateral contraction:
        Bilateral contraction:

33. Internal oblique

    O:

     I:

    N:

    R:

    A: Unilateral contraction:
        Bilateral contraction:

34. Rectus abdominis

    O:

     I:

    N:

    R:

    A:

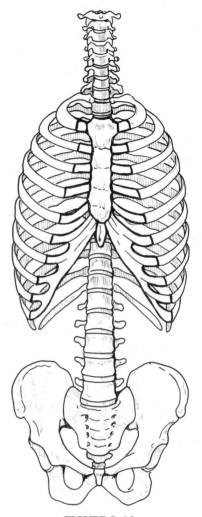

FIGURE 3–13

35. Quadratus lumborum

   O:

    I:

   N:

   R:

  A: Unilateral contraction:

        Bilateral contraction:

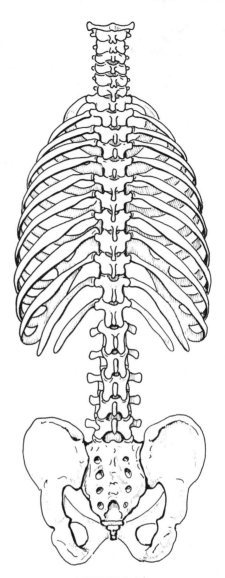

FIGURE 3–14

Neck Muscles

36. Longissimus capitis

    O:
    I:
    N:
    R:
    A:

37. Longissimus cervicis

    O:
    I:
    N:
    R:
    A:

38. Rectus capitis anterior

    O:
    I:
    N:
    R:
    A:

39. Sternocleidomastoid

    O:
    I:
    N:
    R:
    A:

40. Anterior scalenes

    O:
    I:
    N:
    R:
    A:

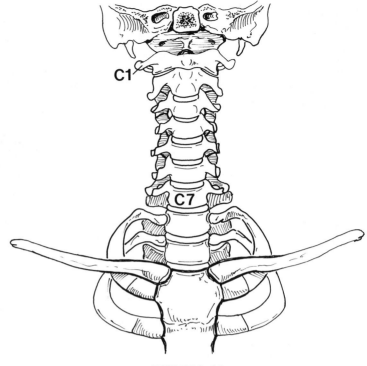

FIGURE 3–15

APPLICATIONS

*41. On a lab partner, palpate the following:

Posterior Aspect of Trunk
Superior nuchal line
Mastoid process
Transverse process of C-1
Spinous process of C-7
Articular pillars of cervical vertebrae
Spinous process of T-3
Inferior angle of scapula
Superior angle of scapula
Medial border of scapula
Lateral border of scapula
Spine of scapula
Posterior superior iliac spines
Ischial tuberosity

Posterior iliac crest
Sacrum
Sacral sulcus
Spinous process of S-2
Spinous process of L-5

Anterior Aspect of Trunk
Coracoid process of scapula
Acromion process of scapula
Suprasternal notch
Anterior and lateral aspect of lower ribs
Anterior superior iliac spines
Iliac crest
Iliac tubercle

*42. You have been palpating while your partner was still. Now have your partner lie on her right side with her hips and knees flexed. Palpate two adjacent spinous processes of the lumbar vertebrae. Continue palpating them while you extend and then flex your partner's lumbar spine. You will do this most easily if your partner is facing you. Put your left fingertips on two adjacent spinous processes. With your right hand and forearm, move your partner's top leg into more flexion. Then move it back into extension. Feel for motion between the spinous processes.

Now have your partner lie prone and stand at her left side. Again, put your left fingertips on two adjacent spinous processes of the lumbar spine. Place the fingers of your right hand anterior to the right anterior superior iliac spine (ASIS) of your partner and raise and lower her right pelvis several times. Feel for motion between the spinous processes. Note that you will not feel a great deal of motion. These are subtle motions that you will be feeling. The inferior spinous process will move a few mm in relation to the superior one.

What is the name of the rotation that you caused in your partner?

*43. Objective measurement of the spine. In groups of three to five, devise a reliable system for objective, quantifiable measurement of trunk range of motion (ROM). On the chart below, note the landmarks selected for measuring each segment and the technique used. For instance, to measure cervical flexion you may choose to use a tape measure (technique) and use the distance from the tip of the chin to the sternal notch (landmarks) at the endpoints of the range of motion. Some standard landmarks exist. One of the purposes of this exercise, however, is to think about and identify stable, logical, and defensible landmarks for motion assessment.

	Flexion/Extension	Lateral Flexion	Rotation
CERVICAL SPINE Landmarks:			
Technique:			
THORACIC SPINE Landmarks:			
Technique:			
LUMBAR SPINE Landmarks:			
Technique:			

*44. Now that you have a scheme for measuring spinal motion, measure each member in your group and record the measurements. What area of the spine appeared to have the greatest flexion? Extension? Side bending? Rotation? How do your measurements relate to your observations from item 15?

*45. In items 43 and 44, you have developed and implemented a method for measuring spinal motion. Could you use the same method to evaluate the normal primary and secondary spinal curves? If you cannot use the method you defined, how could you adapt your method to measure the primary and secondary spinal curves? Measure the primary and secondary spinal curves for each member in your group.

*46. Describe the effects of the following trunk movements on the normal spinal curves of a person standing:

Flexion

Extension or hyperextension

*47. Describe the effects of the following pelvic movements on the normal lumbar curve of a person standing:

Anterior pelvic tilt

Posterior pelvic tilt

*48. Compare the spinal curves of your partner in erect sitting and slouched sitting positions in a chair.

*49. Describe the spinal curves of your partner in the long-sitting position (sitting on a surface with her legs straight out in front of her).

*50. With your partner supine, compare the spinal curves with her legs extended and with her legs flexed at the hip and knee and her feet flat on the supporting surface.

*51. Palpation and observation of muscles. As a general rule, palpate muscles from their origin (or as close as you can get to the origin) to insertion (or as close as you can get to the insertion). Refer to the principles of palpation you identified in item 33 in Chapter 2.

Palpate the following muscles, first on yourself and then on your partner:

Sternocleidomastoid	Scalenes (anterior and middle)
Cervical erector spinae	Rectus abdominis
Thoracic erector spinae	External abdominal oblique
Lumbar erector spinae	Internal abdominal oblique
Splenius capitis	Quadratus lumborum

*52. Demonstrate trunk rotation to the right. Which internal and external obliques are working?

*53. Demonstrate lateral flexion to the right in:

a. An antigravity position. Which internal and external obliques are working? What kind of contraction are they performing? What other muscles might also be working?

b. Standing. Do the muscles acting in this position differ from those working in a? If so, what muscles are now working? What kind of contraction are they performing?

*54. Using Figure 3–16, draw the position of the sacroiliac joint relative to the acetabulum.

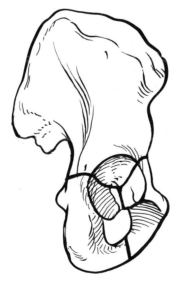

FIGURE 3–16

*55. Describe the effect on the position of the acetabulum of an anterior and a posterior rotation of the ilium on the sacrum. The two positions are represented in Figures 3–17 and 3–18. In each illustration, the original position is represented by a solid line and the rotated position is represented by a broken line. Figure 3–17 represents an anterior rotation of the ilium on the sacrum. Figure 3–18 represents a posterior rotation of the ilium on the sacrum.

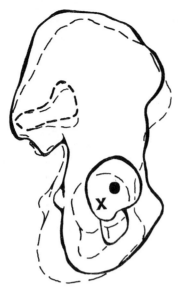

FIGURE 3–17

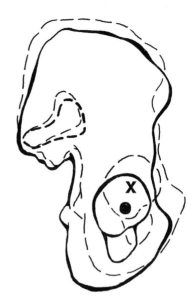

FIGURE 3–18

Effect of anterior rotation

Effect of posterior rotation

*56. For this activity, you will need two identical pieces of paper (3 inches long by ½ inch wide) to represent the lower limb. Use Figure 3-17 (the anteriorly rotated ilium). Apply one piece of paper with the end just touching the axis of motion in the acetabulum with the ilium in neutral (the dot). Apply the second piece of paper with the end just touching the axis of motion in the acetabulum with the ilium rotated (the x). Have both pieces of paper parallel and representing a femur in the anatomical position (vertically aligned on the page). Note that your paper represents the right lower limb.

a. Describe the apparent difference in lower limb length between the two positions.

b. Assume that the left limb has a nonrotated ilium. Describe the effect that you just produced in terms of right lower limb length compared to left lower limb length.

*57. Repeat the procedure, but have the papers represent a lower limb with a flexed hip (horizontally aligned on the page).

    a. Describe the apparent difference in lower limb length between the two positions.

    b. Assume that the left lower limb has a nonrotated ilium. Describe the effect that you just produced in terms of right lower limb length compared to the left.

*58. Repeat the procedure in item 56 on Figure 3–18 (the diagram representing a posteriorly rotated ilium).

    a. Describe the apparent difference in lower limb length between the two positions.

    b. Assume that the left lower limb has a nonrotated ilium. Describe the effect that you just produced in terms of right lower limb length compared to the left lower limb.

*59. Repeat the procedures in item 57 on Figure 3–18 (the diagram representing a posteriorly rotated ilium).

    a. Describe the apparent difference in lower limb length between the two positions.

    b. Assume that the left limb has a nonrotated ilium. Describe the effect that you just produced in terms of right lower limb length compared to the left lower limb.

*60. With a partner, perform the following actions to simulate the motion of the cervical facets during neck motion. The arms and hands of each person represent the facet joint surfaces. In this position, imagine that the bodies of the vertebrae are in front of you. Have one person kneel and hold her arms in the following positions:

    a. Shoulder abduction to about 100°
    b. Elbow in 90° of flexion
    c. Shoulder in 30° of lateral rotation
    d. Forearm pronation

    Have a partner stand behind the kneeler and have her arms in a similar position but with less abduction (70°). The stander's forearms should be parallel to and above the kneeler's forearms. Remember that your arms and hands represent a single bone. Therefore, as you move, do not change their orientation in relation to your body.

    How do the standing person's arms and hands (facet joint surface) move on the kneeling person's arms and hands when the stander bends forward? Make sure that the kneeler does not move her arms. What spinal motion does this represent (remember that the body of the vertebrae is in front of you)? Do the right and left joint surfaces move in the same direction?

*61. How do the standing person's arms and hands (facet joint surface) move on the kneeling person's arms and hands when the stander bends to the right? Remember that the joint capsule will limit significant gapping, but will allow gliding. Make sure the kneeler does not move her arms. What spinal motion does this represent? Do the right and left joint surfaces move in the same direction in relation to each other?

*62. Describe what happens during vertebral rotation. Do the right and left joint surfaces move in the same direction?

*63. Describe what happens during extension. Do the right and left joint surfaces move in the same direction?

NOTE: The relationship of facet motion to segmental motion changes in the various segments of the spine. The observations you have made here are for the cervical area and cannot be generalized for the rest of the spine.

*64. By changing the alignment of your hands and forearms to match the plane of the facets as their orientation changes in each area of the spine, you can get a sense of what motions the facets allow or hinder in the various areas.

a. Have the two partners change the orientation of their facet surfaces to be vertical with forearms pronated. This represents the thoracic spine. What motions are limited and what motions are allowed?

b. Have the two partners change the orientation of their facet surfaces to be vertical with forearms in neutral and the standing subject's arms inside the kneeling subject's arms. This represents the lumbar spine. What motions are limited and what motions are allowed?

*65. For this activity, you will need to palpate at least four subjects; therefore, work in groups of five. During this activity, you will be palpating the relationship of lumbar motion to pelvic motion during forward bending from the standing position. Have your subject standing. With one hand, palpate her lumbar spinous processes. Place the palm of the other hand flat over the sacrum. When your hands are in place, ask the subject to bend forward to touch her toes, and then to return to standing. Repeat this observation on at least four classmates. Remember, you are comparing the amount and sequence of the motion in the lumbar spine and the pelvis. What did you find? At what point in the motion did you begin to feel the pelvis move (early, early middle, middle, late middle, late in the total range of flexion)? This will be the point at which you see your hand, which is on the sacrum, change its plane. Can you make any generalizations?

ANSWERS TO SPINE AND PELVIS

1. Cervical: 7; Thoracic: 12; Lumbar: 5; Sacral: 5; Coccyx: 4

2. Check your text to confirm your information.

3. Convex

4. Cervical: lordotic curve; concave posteriorly; secondary
   Thoracic: kyphotic curve; concave anteriorly; primary
   Lumbar: lordotic curve; concave posteriorly; secondary
   Sacral: kyphotic curve; concave anteriorly; primary

5. Ilium, ischium, pubis

*6. Check your text to confirm your information.

7. Two adjacent vertebrae and the intervening disc for a spinal segment. The spinal nerves exit from the spinal canal through the intervertebral foramen. Note that the spinal cord level and the vertebral level are not the same.

8. Anterior border: vertebral body and disc
   Posterior border: facet joints
   Superior border: pedicle
   Inferior border: pedicle

9. The spinal nerves pass through the intervertebral foramen, so changes in the foramen can have an effect on the spinal nerves.

10. Between L-1 and L-2. Cauda equina.

11. Vertebral body to vertebral body: amphiarthrodial or fibrocartilaginous
    Facet to facet: diarthrodial or synovial
    Pubis to pubis: symphysis or fibrocartilaginous
    Sacrum to ilium: part synovial, part fibrous

12. Vertebral body to vertebral body: tilting and rotation
    Facet to facet: gliding
    Pubis to pubis: slight flexibility of fibrous juncture, but minimal motion allowed
    Sacrum to ilium: gliding, rotation, and gapping

*13. Check your text for accuracy of your information. Have a faculty member or classmate check the accuracy of your placement of the paper and pencil for the planes and axes.

14. Check your text to confirm your information.

*15. There is no "right" answer here. Whatever you found should have been recorded. Individuals will be somewhat different.

16.

Ligament	Location
	Neck
Apical	Tip of the dens to the anterior margin of the foramen magnum
Alar	Two ligaments; from dens laterally to medial aspect of each condyle of occiput
Cruciform	A cross-shaped ligament; attached superiorly to base of occiput near apical ligament, attached inferiorly to posterior surface of body of axis, lateral attachments to tubercles on lateral mass of atlas; transverse portion of ligament is strongest
Tectorial membrane	Posterior surface of body of atlas to base of occiput in front of the foramen magnum
Anterior atlanto-occipital	Anterior arch of atlas to anterior portion of foramen magnum
Posterior atlanto-occipital	Posterior arch of atlas to posterior border of foramen magnum
Ligamentum nuchae	External occipital protuberance to spinous process of C-7
	Thoracic and Lumbar
Supraspinous	Tip of spinous process to tip of spinous process below, from C-7 to sacrum
Interspinous	Length of spinous process to length of spinous process below, primarily in lumbar area
Ligamentum flavum	Posterior aspect of vertebral canal from lamina to lamina from C-2 to sacrum
Posterior longitudinal	Posterior aspect of vertebral body on anterior aspect of vertebral canal from axis to sacrum
Anterior longitudinal	Anterior aspect of vertebral body from axis to sacrum
Intertransverse	Transverse process to transverse process below, primarily in lumbar area
Capsular ligament	Margin of inferior facet of superior vertebra to margin of superior facet of inferior vertebra

17. Check your text to confirm your information.

18. Apical: maintains position of dens and occiput
Alar: limits flexion of head on neck and maintains position of dens
Cruciform: retains dens in close contact with atlas
Tectorial membrane: limits flexion
Anterior atlanto-occipital: limits extension of head on neck
Posterior atlanto-occipital: limits flexion of head on neck
Ligamentum nuchae: limits flexion of head and neck
Supraspinous: limits flexion
Interspinous: limits flexion
Ligamentum flavum: limits flexion
Posterior longitudinal: limits flexion
Anterior longitudinal: limits extension

Intertransverse: limits lateral flexion

Capsular ligament of facet joints: limits gliding of facets

19. Check your text to confirm your information.

20. Both joints move concurrently because the pelvis is a ring, forming a closed kinematic chain. Whenever a movement of the ilium occurs at one end of the ring, movement also occurs at the other end.

21. The superincumbent body weight presses the wedge-shaped sacrum down between the ilia, producing a separating force. The ligaments attaching the sacrum to the ilia are the strongest in the body and become tense from the force. This tension aides in stabilizing the joints in the upright position.

22. Intertransversarii

  O: Transverse process

   I: Transverse process

  N: Dorsal rami of spinal nerve

  R: Posterior to axis for flexion and extension; lateral to axis for side bending

  A: Side bending

23. Interspinales

  O: Spinous process

   I: Spinous process

  N: Dorsal rami of spinal nerves

  R: Posterior to axis for flexion and extension

  A: Extension

24. Semispinalis (spans 3-5 joints)

  O: Transverse process of lower vertebra

   I: Spinous process of higher vertebra

  N: Dorsal rami of spinal nerves

  R: Wraps around the vertical axis; posterior to axis for flexion and extension

  A: Rotation of the body to opposite side; extension if working bilaterally

25. Multifidus (spans 2-3 joints)

  O: Transverse process of lower vertebra

   I: Spinous process of higher vertebra

  N: Dorsal rami of spinal nerve

  R: Posterior to axis for rotation

  A: Rotation of body to opposite side; extension if working bilaterally; side bending to same side

26. Rotatores (spans 1-2 joints)

  O: Transverse process of lower vertebra

   I: Spinous process of higher vertebra

  N: Dorsal rami of spinal nerve

  R: Posterior to axis for rotation

  A: Rotation of the body to opposite side

27. Iliocostalis

  O: Thoracis: tendon of erector spinae; transverse process of lumbar vertebra

      Lumborum: sacrum; spinous process of lumbar and lower thoracic vertebrae; ilium

   I: Thoracis: transverse processes of thoracic vertebrae; ribs

      Lumborum: Lower 6-7 ribs

  N: Dorsal rami of spinal nerve

  R: Posterior to axis for flexion and extension; lateral to axis for side bending

  A: Unilateral contraction: side bending

      Bilateral contraction: extension

28. Longissimus

    O: Transverse processes of lower vertebrae
    I: Transverse processes of higher vertebrae and ribs
    N: Dorsal rami of spinal nerves
    R: Posterior to axis for flexion and extension; lateral to axis for lateral bending
    A: Unilateral contraction: lateral bending
        Bilateral contraction: extension

29. Spinales

    O: Spinous processes of lower vertebrae
    I: Spinous processes of higher vertebrae
    N: Dorsal rami of spinal nerves
    R: Posterior to axis for flexion and extension
    A: Extension

30. Psoas major

    O: Transverse processes and bodies of lumbar vertebrae
    I: Lesser trochanter of femur
    N: Ventral rami of L-2 and L-3
    R: Anterior to axis for flexion and extension
    A: Flexion of femur on pelvis at hip joint

31. Iliacus

    O: Iliac fossa
    I: Lesser trochanter
    N: Femoral n. (L-2, L-3)
    R: Anterior to axis for flexion and extension
    A: Flexion of femur on pelvis at hip joint

32. External oblique

    O: Lower eight ribs
    I: Iliac crest and abdominal aponeurosis
    N: Intercostals (T-8–T-12); iliohypogastric (T-12, L-1); and ilioinguinal (L-1)
    R: Lateral to axis for side bending; anterior to axis for rotation
    A: Unilateral contraction: rotation to opposite side; side bending
        Bilateral contraction: flexion of trunk on pelvis

33. Internal oblique

    O: Inguinal ligament; iliac crest
    I: Linea alba; cartilages of lower ribs
    N: Intercostals (T-8–T-12); iliohypogastric (T-12, L-1); and ilioinguinal (L-1)
    R: Lateral to axis for side bending; anterior to axis for rotation
    A: Unilateral contraction: rotation to same side; side bending
        Bilateral contraction: flexion of trunk on pelvis

34. Rectus abdominis

    O: Crest of pubis
    I: Cartilages of ribs 5, 6, and 7
    N: Intercostal n. (T-7–T-12)
    R: Anterior to axis for flexion and extension
    A: Flexion of trunk on pelvis

35. Quadratus lumborum

    O: Iliolumbar ligament and portion of iliac crest
    I: Last rib and transverse processes of L-1 to L-4
    N: Ventral rami of spinal nerves (T-12, L-1)

R: Lateral to axis for lateral bending

A: Unilateral contraction: lateral bending of trunk on pelvis or elevation of pelvis
Bilateral contraction: extension of lumbar and lower thoracic spine

36. Longissimus capitis

O: Transverse processes of first four or five thoracic vertebrae
I: Mastoid process
N: Dorsal rami of spinal nerves
R: Posterior to axes for flexion and extension and rotation; lateral to axis for side bending
A: Extension; side bending; and rotation of the head to the same side

37. Longissimus cervicis

O: Transverse processes of first four or five thoracic vertebrae
I: Transverse processes of cervical vertebrae
N: Dorsal rami of spinal nerves
R: Posterior to axis for flexion and extension; lateral to axis for side bending
A: Extension and side bending

38. Rectus capitis anterior

O: Lateral mass of atlas
I: Base of occiput anterior to foramen magnum
N: Ventral rami of spinal nerve
R: Anterior to axis for flexion and extension; lateral to axis for side bending
A: Flexion of the head on the neck

39. Sternocleidomastoid

O: Manubrium and medial third of clavicle
I: Mastoid process
N: Spinal accessory nerve (cranial nerve XI)
R: Posterior to axis for flexion and extension of head on neck; anterior to axis of flexion and extension of neck on trunk; lateral to axis for side bending; anterior to axis for rotation
A: Unilateral contraction: extension of head on neck; flexion of neck on trunk; side bending; rotation of head to opposite side
Bilateral contraction: extension of head on neck; flexion of neck on trunk

40. Anterior scalenes

O: Transverse processes of C-3 to C-6
I: Upper surface of first rib
N: Ventral rami of spinal nerves
R: Anterior to axis of flexion and extension of neck on trunk; lateral to axis for side bending; anterior to axis for rotation
A: Unilateral contraction: flexion of neck on trunk; side bending; rotation of head to opposite side
Bilateral contraction: flexion of neck on trunk; elevation of first ribs during inspiration

*41. Have a faculty member confirm your palpations.

*42. Have a faculty member confirm your palpations. Also check with your classmates.
The name of the rotation is left rotation of the lumbar spine because rotation is named by the movement of the superior vertebral body in relation to the inferior vertebral body. In this case, the inferior vertebra rotated right, making the superior vertebra relatively left-rotated.

*43. You may use any landmarks and methods that you can defend. In order to communicate with the rest of the world, though, you should adopt a standardized technique. Consult a goniometry text for standard techniques.

*44. Note that people will be different. A major factor in your measurements that use a tape measure could be the height of the subject.

Generally, the area of the spine with the greatest lateral flexion and rotation is the cervical spine. Extension and flexion are generally greatest in the lumbar spine.

*45. Any method that you choose is acceptable, as long as you can defend it. Chances are that you will not be able to use the same techniques that you developed in item 43.

*46. Flexion tends to increase kyphotic curves and flatten or reverse lordotic curves. Extension or hyperextension tends to decrease or flatten kyphotic curves and increase lordotic curves.

*47. Anterior pelvic tilt increases lumbar lordosis; posterior pelvic tilt decreases lumbar lordosis.

*48. Erect sitting: cervical lordosis, thoracic kyphosis, lumbar lordosis (mild)
Slouched sitting: increased upper cervical lordosis, decreased or reversed lower cervical lordosis, increased thoracic kyphosis, decreased or reversed lumbar lordosis.

*49. Cervical: usually unaffected from normal
Thoracic: unaffected or mildly increased kyphosis
Lumbar: usually decreased lordosis caused by tightness in hamstrings

*50. Supine with legs extended tends to increase lumbar lordosis, especially if the individual's hip flexors are tight. Flexing the knees slackens the hip flexors so that the lumbar spine will not be pulled into increased lordosis.

*51. Have a faculty member check the accuracy of your palpations.

*52. The left external and right internal abdominal obliques will cause rotation to the right.

*53. a. To flex laterally to the right against gravity requires the internal and external abdominal obliques on the right side to contract.
   b. To flex laterally to the right in standing requires the left internal *and* external abdominal obliques to contract eccentrically to control the motion of right side bending. Gravity is causing the motion.

*54. See Figure 3–19.

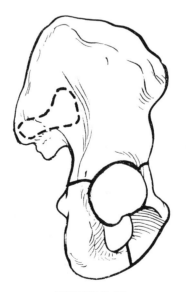

FIGURE 3–19

*55. Anterior rotation causes the acetabulum to move distally and posteriorly; posterior rotation causes the acetabulum to move superiorly and anteriorly.

*56. With an anteriorly rotated ilium, the lower limb with an extended hip appears longer than when the ilium is not rotated. The right lower limb would appear longer than the left.

*57. With an anteriorly rotated ilium, the lower limb with a flexed hip and extended knee appears shorter than when the ilium is not rotated. The right lower limb would appear shorter than it did in the hip-extended position.

*58. With a posteriorly rotated ilium, the lower limb with an extended hip appears shorter than when the ilium is not rotated. The right lower limb would appear shorter than the left.

*59. With a posteriorly rotated ilium, the lower limb with a flexed hip and extended knee appears longer than when the ilium is not rotated. The right lower limb would appear longer than it did in the hip-extended position.

*60. The standing person bending forward represents cervical flexion, and the facets of the superior vertebra glide forward over the facets of the inferior vertebra in this motion.

*61. Bending to the right represents right lateral flexion, and the right facet of the superior vertebra glides backward while the left glides forward over the facets of the inferior vertebra.

*62. The same facet motions that occurred in lateral flexion (item 61) occur during rotation in the cervical spine.

*63. During extension, both the right and left facets of the superior vertebra glide backward over the facets of the inferior vertebra.

*64. a. Flexion and extension are more limited by the facet joints than rotation and side bending. The rib cage is a major factor limiting thoracic motion and is unrelated to the alignment of the facets.
    b. Side bending and rotation are more limited than flexion and extension.

*65. Flexion of the trunk from the standing position (as in touching the toes) is usually composed of flexion of the lumbar spine and an anterior tilt of the pelvis on the femur. The return to standing is the reverse of these motions. Lumbosacral rhythm refers to the proportion of motion that is at the hip versus the lumbar spine. In going from erect standing to a 90° angle (the trunk parallel to the floor), the lumbar spine is responsible for approximately 45° of flexion and the pelvis tilting on the femur at the hip is responsible for the other 45° of motion. You probably noted some variations from this general rule.

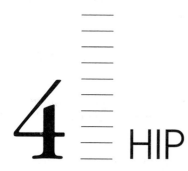

4 HIP

OSTEOLOGY OF THE HIP

The bones to include when considering the hip joint are the pelvis and the femur.

Pelvis

1. Label the following parts of the pelvis on Figure 4-1:

   Iliac crest
   Anterior superior iliac spine
   Anterior inferior iliac spine
   Posterior superior iliac spine
   Greater sciatic notch

   Lesser sciatic notch
   Ischial spine
   Ischial tuberosity
   Pubic crest

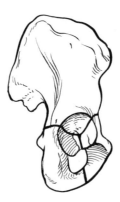

FIGURE 4-1

2. During development, what three bones come together and fuse in the acetabulum to form one hemipelvis? (See Figure 4-1.)

Femur

3. Label the following parts of the femur on Figure 4-2:

Head	Lesser trochanter
Neck	Adductor tubercle
Shaft	Linea aspera
Greater trochanter	Condyles

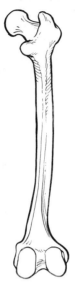

FIGURE 4–2

4. On the diagram of the femur in Figure 4-2, outline the angle of inclination of the femur.

   a. How many degrees of inclination does the femur in the diagram show? (Hint: Use your goniometer.)
   b. Is this normal for an adult femur?

5. In what view would you need to place a disarticulated skeletal femur in order to visualize the torsion in the shaft?

6. What parts of the femur do femoral anteversion and femoral retroversion refer to? Define anteversion and retroversion of the femur.

ARTHROLOGY OF THE HIP

The joints to consider when studying the hip region include the sacroiliac joint, the symphysis pubis, and the hip joint itself. Note: The sacroiliac joint and symphysis pubis were addressed in Chapter 3.

Hip Joint (Femoroacetabular Joint)

7. What type of joint is the hip joint?

8. What motions are available at the hip?

9. Draw the following ligaments of the hip joint on Figures 4–3 to 4–5. Be sure to indicate the main direction of the fibers of each ligament.

   Iliofemoral ligament
   Pubofemoral ligament
   Ischiofemoral ligament

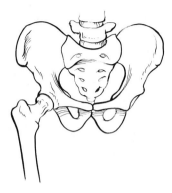

FIGURE 4–3

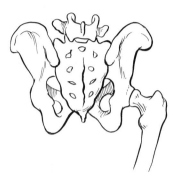

FIGURE 4–4

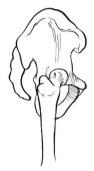

FIGURE 4–5

10. Considering the direction of the fibers of each of the ligaments drawn in item 9, what hip motion would each ligament restrain?

   a. Iliofemoral
   b. Pubofemoral
   c. Ischiofemoral

11. What is another name for the iliofemoral ligament?

*12. On a subject who is lying supine, place the left hip in the open-packed position and then in the close-packed position. Verify the position by movement of the joint.

13. Which of the bursae directly associated with the anatomy of the hip is the most superficial?

*14. Palpate the following items on several different subjects:

   Anterior superior iliac spine   Greater trochanter
   Iliac crest   Posterior superior iliac spine
   Iliac tubercle   Ischial tuberosity
   Femoral triangle   Posterior spinous process of L-5
   Femoral pulse   Sacral sulcus

MYOLOGY OF THE HIP

Use the following muscle sheets to aid in learning the origins, insertions, and innervations of the hip muscles. For each muscle named, draw in the muscle on the sketch and complete the indicated information on the outline. The first two muscles have completed information as examples. The following abbreviations apply throughout the muscle sheets:

O: Origin of muscle
I: Insertion of muscle
N: Innervation (both peripheral nerve and spinal levels)
R: Relationship of muscle to axis of motion
A: Action of muscle

15. Gluteus maximus

O: Lateral lip of iliac crest; posterior surfaces of lower part of sacrum and side of coccyx; posterior surface of sacrotuberous ligament
I: Iliotibial band of fascia lata over greater trochanter and the gluteal tuberosity of the femur
N: Inferior gluteal n. (L-5, S-1, S-2)
R: Posterior to axis for hip flexion and extension; posterior and lateral to axis for hip rotation
A: Extension and lateral rotation of the femur at the hip

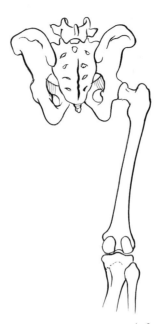

FIGURE 4–6

16. Gluteus medius

O: Outer ilium and iliac crest
I: Lateral aspect of greater trochanter of the femur
N: Superior gluteal n. (L-4, L-5, S-1)
R: Lateral (or superior) to axis for abduction and adduction
A: Abduction of the femur at the hip

17. Gluteus minimus

O: Posterior and outer surface of ilium
I: Greater trochanter of the femur (anterior aspect)
N:
R: Lateral (or superior) to axis for abduction and adduction; anterior for rotation
A: Abduction and medial rotation of the femur at the hip

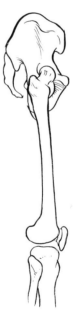

FIGURE 4–7

18. Semitendinosus

    O: Ischial tuberosity

    I: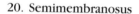

    N: Tibial portion of sciatic n. (L-4, L-5, S-1, S-2)

    R: Posterior to axes for both hip flexion and extension and knee flexion and extension; medial to axis for tibial rotation

    A: Extension of the femur at the hip; flexion and medial rotation of the tibia at the knee

19. Biceps femoris

    O: Long head:
       Short head:

    I: Lateral aspect of head of fibula; lateral epicondyle of tibia

    N: Tibial portion of sciatic n. (L-5, S-1, S-2)

    R: Posterior to axes for both hip flexion and extension and knee flexion and extension; lateral to axis for tibial rotation

    A:

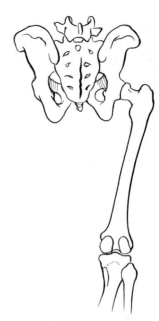

FIGURE 4–6

20. Semimembranosus

    O: Ischial tuberosity

    I:

    N:

    R: Posterior to axes for hip flexion and extension and knee flexion and extension; medial to axis for tibial rotation

    A: Extension of the femur at the hip; flexion and medial rotation of the tibia at the knee

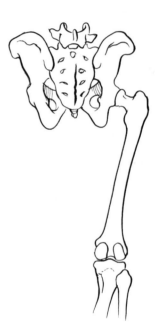

FIGURE 4–6

21. Adductor magnus

    O: Inferior surface of ischium; anterior surface of pubic ramus

    I:

    N: Obturator n. (and some fibers from sciatic n.) (L-2, L-3, L-4, L-5, S-1)

    R: Medial (or inferior) to axis for abduction and adduction; anterior to axis for flexion and extension (upper fibers); posterior to axis for flexion and extension (lower fibers)

    A:

22. Adductor brevis

    O:

    I:

    N:

    R: Medial and inferior to axis for abduction and adduction

    A: Adduction of the femur at the hip

23. Adductor longus

    O: Anterior pubis between crest and symphysis

    I: Linea aspera of femur

    N: Obturator n. (L-2, L-3, L-4)

    R:

    A:

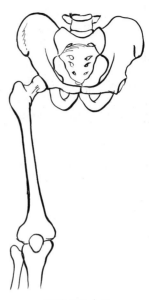

FIGURE 4–8

24. Pectineus

    O:

    I: Pectineal line of femur

    N:

    R:

    A: Adduction of femur at the hip; flexion of femur at the hip if the femur is laterally rotated; lateral rotation of femur at the hip

25. Gracilis

    O: Arch of symphysis pubis

    I:

    N:

    R: Medial (or inferior) to axis for abduction and adduction; posterior to axis for flexion and extension of tibia at the knee; anterior and medial to axis for rotation of the tibia at the knee

    A: Adduction of the femur at the hip; flexion and medial rotation of the tibia at the knee

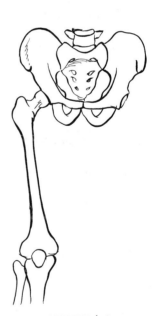

FIGURE 4–8

26. Sartorius

    O:

    I: Anteromedial surface of proximal tibia

    N:

    R: Anterior to axis for flexion and extension; anterior and wraps medially around axis for rotation

    A:

27. Obturator externus

    O:

    I:

    N:

    R: Posterior and wraps laterally around axis for rotation

    A: Lateral rotation of the femur at the hip

28. Obturator internus

    O: Obturator foramen (inner margin); superior aspect of greater sciatic foramen

    I:

    N: Nerve to obturator internus (L-5, S-1, S-2)

    R:

    A: Lateral rotation of the femur at the hip

29. Quadratus femoris

    O:

    I: Intertubercular line of femur

    N: Nerve to quadratus femoris (L-4, L-5, S-1, S-2)

    R:

    A:

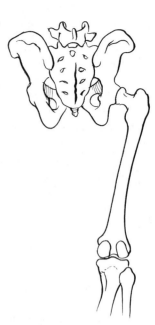

FIGURE 4–6

30. Piriformis

    O:

    I:

    N: Nerve to piriformis (L-5, S-1, S-2)

    R:

    A: Lateral rotation (and some abduction) of the femur at the hip

31. Gemellus inferior

    O:

    I:

    N: Branch of nerve to quadratus femoris (L-4, L-5, S-1, S-2)

    R: Posterior and superior to the axis for lateral rotation

    A:

32. Gemellus superior

    O: Outer surface of ischial spine

    I:

    N:

    R:

    A: Lateral rotation (and some abduction) of the femur at the hip

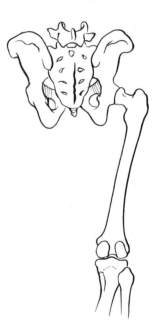

FIGURE 4–6

33. Tensor fascia lata

   O:

   I: Iliotibial tract. (Note that this muscle does not
     attach directly to the bone.)

   N:

   R:

   A:

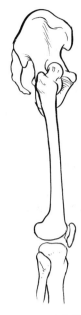

FIGURE 4–7

34. Iliopsoas

   O: Iliacus: superior iliac fossa; inner lip of iliac crest;

     base of sacrum

     Psoas major: transverse processes of all lumbar
     vertebrae; sides of bodies and discs of last thoracic
     and all lumbar vertebrae

   I:

   N:

   R:

   A:

35. Rectus femoris

   O:

   I:

   N:

   R:

   A:

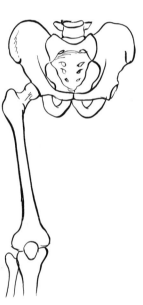

FIGURE 4–8

APPLICATIONS

*36. Select a subject dressed in shorts. Have the subject perform the combined action of adduction of the femur at the hip with flexion and medial rotation of the tibia at the knee.

    a. Palpate the muscle primarily responsible for this combined action.

    b. How is this muscle affected by knee flexion during hip adduction?

    c. Demonstrate on a laboratory partner how you would test for tightness in this muscle.

*37. During normal gait, the gluteus medius mainly works in reverse action. Demonstrate a gait pattern associated with a weak or absent right gluteus medius.

    a. Discuss how a patient may reduce the torque produced by gravitational force on the center of mass in order to compensate for weakness of the gluteus medius.

    b. On Figure 4-9, draw the vectors showing the relationship of forces acting on the hip joint during single limb support.

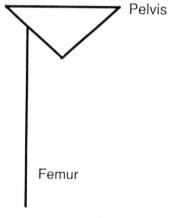

FIGURE 4–9

*38. In a standing position, demonstrate the effect of bilateral tight iliopsoas on hip joint position.

    a. Now demonstrate the same muscle tightness in the supine position.

    b. Describe the position of the lumbar spine when lying supine with thighs on the table and demonstrating the effect of tight iliopsoas.

    c. Develop a kinesiological rationale for what you have described in b.

*39. Which muscles form a force couple by producing forces anterior and posterior to the hip joint to cause a posterior pelvic tilt?

    a. In standing, assume a posteriorly tilted pelvis.

    b. Describe the movement of the hip joint as you performed the tilt and the position of the lumbar spine once you have assumed the position.

    c. Describe how, in a closed kinematic chain, movement of the pelvis on the hip affects the posture of the lumbar spine.

    d. What type of action is movement of the pelvis on the femur?

*40. Position your partner's lower extremity so that passive insufficiency of the hamstrings limits the range of motion of flexion of the femur at the hip.

*41. Position your partner's lower extremity so that passive insufficiency of the rectus femoris limits the range of motion of extension of the femur at the hip.

42. a. Discuss the interaction of the hip and knee joint positions to avoid active insufficiency when the hamstrings or the rectus femoris are actively contracting. In your discussion, include the effects of joint position on active insufficiency of each of the muscles.

    b. Discuss the interaction of the hip and knee joint positions to avoid passive insufficiency when the hamstrings or the rectus femoris are tight. In your discussion, include the effects of joint position on passive insufficiency of each of the muscles.

    c. Describe the elegance of normal lower extremity movement that avoids active and passive insufficiency by maintaining a favorable length-tension relationship in the hamstrings and rectus femoris. Elegance means efficiency and simplicity in movement.

*43. Devise and perform a method of stretching the gluteus maximus without interference from the hamstrings.

44. Describe the motion resulting from an active contraction of the gluteus maximus without concurrent contraction of the gluteus minimus. Explain your answer.

*45. Perform a flexibility test for the hip flexors that differentiates between tightness of the iliopsoas and tightness of the rectus femoris.

46. An athlete has a bruise over the anterior superior iliac spine (ASIS). What active muscle contractions could be most painful?

47. Position your partner to muscle-test the iliopsoas so that there will be minimal contribution from the rectus femoris to the strength of the movement.

48. The lesser trochanter of the femur is avulsed from the shaft of the femur as a large jagged fragment that retains its muscle attachment(s). What reverse action could be particularly painful? Explain your answer.

*49. Mimic the standing posture of an individual with bilateral paralysis of the gluteus maximus. What is the biomechanical explanation for the posture you assumed; that is, how does this posture compensate for paralyzed gluteus maximus muscles?

*50. While standing on your right lower limb, rotate your pelvis to the right (clockwise) in the horizontal plane. See Figure 4–10 below. In what *rotated* position is the right femur at the hip at the end of the rotation?

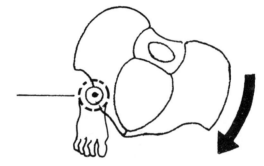

FIGURE 4–10

*51. While standing on both lower limbs, rotate your pelvis to the left (counterclockwise). In what *rotated* position is each femur at the hip at the end of the pelvic rotation?

*52. Stand on your right lower limb on a step stool. This will allow the left limb to swing freely below the pelvis. Start with your left hip extended and the knee flexed (your foot should be well behind you). Now, swing the entire limb forward with flexion of the femur at the hip and extension of the tibia at the knee. *Actively slow* the rate of swing at the hip and the knee before the end range is reached.

  a. What muscles did you use to use to slow the rate of swing at the hip? At the knee?

  b. What type of contraction did the muscles perform to slow the swinging limb?

*53. Step slowly down from the stool. Concentrate on which hip muscles seem to be working the most in the right hip. Which muscles are they and what type of contraction are they performing?

*54. Give your right hip a rest and stand on the left, but stand on it with your trunk erect, knee straight, and hip flexed as much as possible (which will not be much). Your left foot should be slightly forward and you will feel your body weight in the heel.

   a. What hip muscles are responsible for maintaining this position?

   b. Why is it hard to maintain this position?

*55. The most common direction for the hip to dislocate is posteriorly. Examine a skeleton and determine the combined hip position that can lead to a dislocated hip, particularly if the joint is weakened as in total joint replacement surgery.

   a. Considering only the bony anatomy in the erect skeleton, where would you guess the direction of dislocation to be?

   b. Why is it not that direction?

   c. What is the effect of posterior hip dislocation on gluteus medius length, and what would the resulting gait deviation be? Why?

ANSWERS TO HIP

1. Check your text and have a faculty member confirm your information.

2. The three bones that fuse to comprise the pelvis are the ilium, ischium, and pubis.

3. Check your text and have a faculty member confirm your information.

4. The angle of inclination is between the neck and shaft of the femur in the frontal plane.
   a. 122° of inclination
   b. Yes

5. Position the femur so that you are viewing it along the long axis and so that the femoral condyles are parallel to a reference line. The easiest way to accomplish these position criteria is to lay the femur on a tabletop with the anterior surface up and both condyles in contact with the tabletop.

6. Femoral anteversion and retroversion refer to the orientation of the neck of the femur to the shaft. The orientation is in the horizontal plane. Anteversion is a twisting of the shaft so that the neck and head of the femur point more anteriorly than normally in respect to the shaft. Retroversion has the head and neck pointing more posteriorly than normally.

7. The hip joint is a diarthrodial ball-and-socket joint.

8. Flexion and extension; adduction and abduction; medial and lateral rotation; circumduction.

9. Check your text and have a faculty member confirm your information.

10. a. Iliofemoral ligament restricts extension.
    b. Pubofemoral ligament restricts extension and abduction.
    c. Ischiofemoral ligament restricts extension.

11. Another name for the iliofemoral ligament is the Y ligament of Bigelow.

12. The open-packed position of the hip is flexion and lateral rotation of the femur at the hip. The close-packed position is extension and medial rotation of the femur at the hip. The joint will be flexible in the open-packed position and tight in the close-packed position.

13. The most superficial bursa of the hip is the trochanteric bursa between the attachment of the gluteus maximus on the iliotibial tract and the greater trochanter.

14. *The standard kinesiology, anatomy, or muscle-testing text should allow completion of this activity. Faculty confirmation of the palpations is helpful.

15. Gluteus maximus: answers given in text.

16. Gluteus medius: answers given in text.

17. Gluteus minimus

    O: Posterior and outer surface of ilium
    I: Greater trochanter of the femur (anterior aspect)
    N: Superior gluteal n. (L-4, L-5, S-1)
    R: Lateral (or superior) to axis for abduction and adduction; anterior to axis for rotation
    A: Abduction and medial rotation of the femur at the hip

18. Semitendinosus

    O: Ischial tuberosity
    I: Anteromedial surface of proximal tibia
    N: Tibial portion of sciatic n. (L-4, L-5, S-1, S-2)
    R: Posterior to axes for both hip flexion and extension and knee flexion and extension; medial to axis for tibial rotation
    A: Extension of the femur at the hip; flexion and medial rotation of the tibia at the knee

19. Biceps femoris

    O: Long head: Ischial tuberosity
       Short head: Linea aspera
    I: Lateral aspect of head of fibula; lateral epicondyle of tibia
    N: Tibial portion of sciatic n. (L-5, S-1, S-2)
    R: Posterior to axes for both hip flexion and extension and knee flexion and extension; lateral to axis for tibial rotation
    A: Extension of the femur at the hip; flexion and lateral rotation of the tibia at the knee

20. Semimembranosus

    O: Ischial tuberosity
    I: Posteromedial aspect of medial epicondyle of tibia
    N: Tibial portion of sciatic n. (L-4, L-5, S-1, S-2)
    R: Posterior to axes for both hip flexion and extension and knee flexion and extension; medial to axis for tibial rotation
    A: Extension of the femur at the hip; flexion and medial rotation of the tibia at the knee

21. Adductor magnus

    O: Inferior surface of ischium; anterior surface of pubic ramus
    I: Linea aspera; adductor tubercle
    N: Obturator n. and some fibers from sciatic n. (L-2, L-3, L-4, L-5, S-1)
    R: Medial (or inferior) to axis for abduction and adduction; anterior to axis for flexion and extension (upper fibers); posterior to axis for flexion and extension (lower fibers)
    A: Adduction of the femur at the hip; flexion of the femur at the hip if femur is laterally rotated; extension of the femur at the hip if femur is medially rotated

22. Adductor brevis

    O: Inferior ramus of pubis
    I: Femur, distal to lesser trochanter and continuing to linea aspera
    N: Obturator n. (L-2, L-3, L-4)
    R: Medial and inferior to axis for abduction and adduction
    A: Adduction of the femur at the hip

23. Adductor longus

    O: Anterior pubis between crest and symphysis
    I: Linea aspera of femur
    N: Obturator n. (L-2, L-3, L-4)
    R: Medial and inferior to axis for abduction and adduction; anterior to axis for flexion and extension
    A: Adduction of the femur at the hip; flexion of the femur at the hip

24. Pectineus

    O: Pubic tubercle
    I: Pectineal line of femur
    N: Femoral n. (L-2, L-3, L-4)
    R: Medial and inferior to axis for abduction and adduction; anterior to axis for flexion and extension
    A: Adduction of the femur at the hip; flexion of the femur at the hip if the femur is laterally rotated; lateral rotation of the femur at the hip

25. Gracilis

    O: Arch of symphysis pubis
    I: Anteromedial surface of proximal tibia
    N: Obturator n. (L-2, L-3, L-4)
    R: Medial (or inferior) to axis for abduction and adduction; posterior to axis for flexion and extension of tibia at the knee; anterior and medial to axis for rotation of the tibia at the knee
    A: Adduction of the femur at the hip; flexion and medial rotation of the tibia at the knee

26. Sartorius

    O: Anterior superior iliac spine
    I: Anteromedial surface of proximal tibia
    N: Femoral n. (L-2, L-3, L-4)
    R: Anterior to axis for flexion and extension; anterior and wraps medially around axis for rotation
    A: Flexion and lateral rotation of the femur at the hip

27. Obturator externus

    O: Medial side of obturator foramen; medial outer surface of obturator membrane; pubic and ischial rami
    I: Posterior surface of femoral neck
    N: Obturator n. (L-3, L-4)
    R: Posterior and wraps around axis for rotation
    A: Lateral rotation of the femur at the hip

28. Obturator internus

    O: Obturator foramen (inner margin); superior aspect of greater sciatic foramen
    I: Through lesser sciatic notch; proceeds to medial surface of greater trochanter
    N: Nerve to obturator internus (L-5, S-1, S-2)
    R: Posterior to the axis for rotation
    A: Lateral rotation of the femur at the hip

29. Quadratus femoris

    O: Ischial tuberosity
    I: Intertubercular line of femur
    N: Nerve to quadratus femoris (L-4, L-5, S-1, S-2)
    R: Posterior to the axis for rotation
    A: Lateral rotation of the femur at the hip

30. Piriformis

    O: Anterior sacrum and greater sciatic notch
    I: Upper portion of greater trochanter
    N: Nerve to piriformis (L-5, S-1, S-2)
    R: Posterior to the axis for rotation
    A: Lateral rotation (and some abduction) of the femur at the hip

31. Gemellus inferior

    O: Ischial tuberosity
    I: Greater trochanter
    N: Branch of nerve to quadratus femoris (L-4, L-5, S-1, S-2)
    R: Posterior and superior to the axis for rotation
    A: Lateral rotation (and some abduction) of the femur at the hip

32. Gemellus superior

    O: Outer surface of ischial spine
    I: Greater trochanter
    N: Branch of nerve to obturator internus (L-5, S-1, S-2)
    R: Posterior and wraps around axis for rotation
    A: Lateral rotation (and some abduction) of the femur at the hip

33. Tensor fascia lata

    O: Anterior superior iliac spine
    I: Iliotibial tract (note that this muscle does not attach directly to bone)
    N: Superior gluteal n. (L-4, L-5, S-1)
    R: Anterior to axis for flexion and extension; anterior and lateral to axis for rotation
    A: Flexion of femur at the hip; medial rotation of femur at the hip

34. Iliopsoas

    O: Iliacus: superior iliac fossa, inner lip of iliac crest; base of sacrum
       Psoas major: transverse processes of all lumbar vertebrae; sides of bodies and discs of last thoracic and all lumbar vertebrae
    I: Iliacus: tendon of the psoas major; distal to the lesser trochanter
       Psoas major: lesser trochanter
    N: Iliacus: branches from the femoral n. (L-1, L-2, L-3, L-4)
       Psoas major: branches directly from the lumbar plexus (L-1, L-2, L-3, L-4)
    R: Anterior to the axis for flexion and extension
    A: Flexion of the femur at the hip

35. Rectus femoris

    O: Anterior inferior iliac spine

    I: Base of the patella and from there to the tibial tuberosity

    N: Femoral n. (L-2, L-3, L-4)

    R: Anterior to the axes for flexion and extension of the femur at the hip and flexion and extension of the tibia at the knee

    A: Flexion of the femur at the hip and extension of the tibia at the knee

*36. The gracilis adducts the hip and produces slight flexion and medial rotation of the tibia at the knee.

    a. Consult your texts for palpation locations and confirm them with a faculty member.

    b. The muscle is weakened by knee flexion during adduction of the femur at the hip. Since it shortens with both movements, it becomes actively insufficient when both movements occur simultaneously.

    c. The learner should find a method to simultaneously abduct the hip and extend the knee. This position will produce passive insufficiency in the muscle. This exercise can assist the learner in acquiring the skill of differentiating between tightness in one-joint and two-joint muscles, for example, tightness in the one-joint adductors (abduction with knees flexed) and the two-joint adductor (as above).

*37. With weakness or paralysis of the right gluteus medius, there is an exaggerated drop of the pelvis on the left side during stance on the right.

    a. Once the learners have tried this activity, a visual representation of this gait pattern is likely to be necessary to provide the learners with a reference from which to reproduce the gait pattern. This can be provided by the faculty, a fellow student with clinical experience, or videotape. Demonstrate how the patient may produce a lateral lurch of the trunk over the stance limb.

    b.

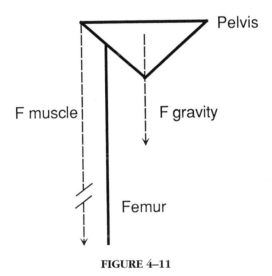

FIGURE 4–11

38. The learner assumes a position of increased lumbar lordosis, assuming that the thoracic spine remains vertical. The exercise is meant to reinforce the effect of a tight iliopsoas muscle on trunk posture.

    a. and b. Now, in the supine position, the femurs may rise off the table to hide the effect on the lumbar spine. If not, then the increased lordosis can be seen easily with increased space between the lumbar spine and the table.

    c. Since the proximal attachment for the iliopsoas is on the ilium and lumbar spine, if the muscle shortens with the femur remaining stationary, the pelvis and lumbar spine move anteriorly (flex) at the hip. This is anterior pelvic tilt and increases the lumbar lordosis.

*39. Anteriorly, the abdominals attach to the pubic rami; posteriorly, the hamstrings attach to the ischial tuberosity and the gluteus maximus attaches to the sacrum. Together, they produce posterior pelvic tilt when moving the pelvis on the femur (closed kinematic chain).

    a. Again, a visual demonstration may be necessary to allow the learners to successfully reproduce the posterior pelvic tilt.

    b. The anterior angle of the hip joint opens during a posterior pelvic tilt; thus this is extension of the hip, which decreases the lumbar lordosis.

    c. In a closed kinematic chain, most easily seen with the femurs stationary, movement of the pelvis at the hip simultaneously produces movement at the lumbar spine. Anterior pelvic tilt produces increased lumbar lordosis (extension of the lumbar spine), and posterior pelvic tilt produces decreased lumbar lordosis (flexion of the lumbar spine). A visual reproduction of this action with an articulated skeletal spine is usually helpful in the explanation.

    d. Anterior and posterior pelvic tilt are examples of reverse actions with the proximal attachment moving and the distal attachment stationary.

*40. This is to demonstrate the interdependence of joint action on a two-joint muscle. This item can also be used to examine the effect of tight hamstrings on low back posture. The effect will be emphasized if the knee is straight during a passive straight leg raise. This activity may lead into a discussion of what postural changes to look for when examining for hamstring tightness. It can also facilitate a discussion of the larger concept of a tight or contracting muscle producing postural effects at remote joints.

*41. The same issues as addressed in item 40 are reinforced here. The hip must be extended with the knee flexed.

42. a. During strong active contraction of the hamstrings in their function as hip extensors, the concurrent joint movements are knee extension with hip extension. With contraction of the rectus femoris in its role as a hip flexor, the concurrent joint movements are knee flexion with hip flexion. In each of these movements, the knee joint motion compensates for the shortening of the muscle at the hip; that is, as the hamstrings shorten during hip extension, they are being lengthened at the knee by knee extension.

    b. Since the hamstrings cross the hip and the knee posteriorly, tightness in the hamstrings will limit hip flexion and knee extension. The maximum effect can be seen if these movements are produced simultaneously, as in a straight leg raise. Since the rectus femoris crosses the hip and knee anteriorly, the reciprocal relationship is represented.

    c. There is a relationship between the rectus femoris and the hamstrings in action and in joint position for active and passive insufficiency. The combined joint action that avoids *passive insufficiency* in the *hamstrings* during hip flexion (flexion of the knee with flexion of the hip) also avoids *active insufficiency* in the *rectus femoris* in its function as a hip flexor. The position producing active insufficiency for one (thus to be avoided) produces passive insufficiency for the other, so postures that avoid active insufficiency for one muscle simultaneously avoid passive insufficiency for the other.

*43. Several solutions are undoubtedly possible. One option is to lie supine, flex the knee, and flex the hip. Knee flexion slackens the hamstrings; thus any muscle tightness felt in hip flexion with the knee flexed is most likely tightness in the gluteus maximus.

44. The result of a contraction of the gluteus maximus without contraction of the gluteus minimus would be extension with lateral rotation of the femur at the hip. The medial rotation provided by a simultaneous contraction of the gluteus minimus neutralizes the lateral rotation component of the gluteus maximus, allowing pure extension.

*45. The critical item here is to stabilize the pelvis while measuring unilateral passive extension of the femur at the hip; once with the knee flexed and once with the knee extended. This activity is meant to reinforce principles of two-joint muscles, as well as demonstrate the clinical significance of the effect two-joint versus one-joint muscles have on joint motion.

46. Since the tensor fascia lata and sartorius attach to the ASIS, their actions will be most painful.

*47. To limit the participation of the rectus femoris in active flexion of the femur at the hip, put the limb in a position in which the rectus femoris is at an inefficient length for contraction (is actively insufficient), then ask for an active hip flexion contraction. The muscle left to perform the motion is mainly the iliopsoas.

48. The reverse action that is painful is coming to a sitting position from a lying one because the iliopsoas pulls its attachment on the lesser trochanter. This attachment is now a jagged fragment being pulled by the muscle contraction into the pelvic cavity.

*49. The position assumed will be with both hips in extension past 0°. This places the line of gravity for the trunk behind the hip joint; thus gravity produces a posterior moment of rotation at the hip. This force produces extension of the pelvis at the hip, which had been the role of the gluteus maximus. The iliofemoral ligament provides the main resistance to stop further extension, but the pubofemoral and ischiofemoral ligaments of the hip also become tight as the joint moves toward the close-packed position.

*50. The hip ends up in medial rotation; that is, the femur is medially rotated on the pelvis.

*51. The left femur is now medially rotated at the hip and the right femur is laterally rotated at the hip.

*52. a. The muscles used were the gluteus maximus at the hip and hamstrings at the hip and the knee.
    b. They performed an eccentric contraction. This information will be specifically utilized in Chapter 12.

*53. The most active hip muscles were the extensors (gluteus maximus and hamstrings) performing an eccentric contraction.

*54. a. In order to maintain the flexed hip position against gravity, the hip extensors must be active. We will need this information again in Chapter 12.
    b. It was difficult to maintain because the line of gravity of the body was falling behind the base of support.

*55. If you flex, adduct, and medially rotate the femur at the hip, the head of the femur becomes uncovered by the acetabulum posteriorly. This is the position of dislocation, especially for patients who have had total hip replacement surgery.

    a. Anteriorly
    b. The anterior ligaments are the strongest.
    c. The gluteus medius will be shortened. This produces active insufficiency in the muscle and weakens it. The gait pattern typical for a weak gluteus medius is the Trendelenburg pattern or the gluteus medius limp or lurch.

5 KNEE

OSTEOLOGY OF THE KNEE

1. On Figures 5-1 to 5-3, label the following bony landmarks and place an asterisk by those that are palpable.

Lateral epicondyle, femur
Patellar facet for medial femoral condyle
Medial condyle of tibia
Tubercles of intercondylar eminence
Lateral condyle of tibia
Head of fibula
Tibial tuberosity
Base of patella

Lateral condyle, femur
Medial epicondyle, femur
Medial condyle, femur
Adductor tubercle
Patellar surface of femur
Patellar facet for lateral femoral condyle
Apex of patella

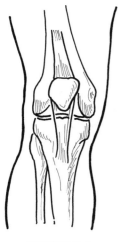

FIGURE 5–1

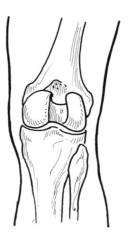

FIGURE 5–2

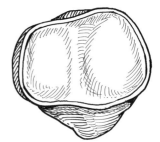

FIGURE 5–3

2. Describe the posterior surface of the patella.

3. From an anterior view of a vertical femur, describe the asymmetry of the femoral condyles. What significance does this asymmetry hold for knee posture?

4. In the space below, draw an anterior view and a superior view of the tibial plateau of the left tibia, including the menisci. Do not include ligaments. Shade the menisci along their areas of attachment.

ARTHROLOGY OF THE KNEE

5. On Figures 5-4 and 5-5, label the following soft tissue structures with the appropriate letter. Draw in the patellar ligament as if it were dissected from the patella but still attached inferiorly.

   a. Medial (tibial) collateral ligament
   b. Lateral (fibular) collateral ligament
   c. Medial meniscus
   d. Lateral meniscus
   e. Anterior cruciate ligament
   f. Posterior cruciate ligament

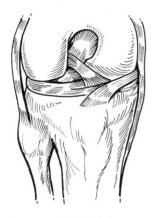

FIGURE 5–4

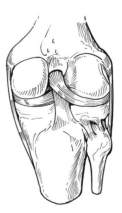

FIGURE 5–5

*6. On a subject, palpate the following soft tissue structures around the knee.

Joint line (medial and lateral)
Medial collateral ligament
Lateral collateral ligament

HINT: It is easier to find the joint line if the tibia is passively moved on the femur while you are palpating the area. It is also easier to find the collateral ligaments when you stress the ligament with the joint slightly flexed.

7. List the major articular surfaces and soft tissue structures residing within the articular capsule of the knee. Examine the cruciate ligaments for their relationship to the main articular capsule.

8. The knee is not a pure hinge joint. Why?

*9. The intrajoint actions of spin, roll, and glide are most easily demonstrated in the movements of the knee joint. Examine the chapter on the knee joint in your kinesiology text. Use an anatomical model to demonstrate and explain the following:

a. How gliding interacts with rolling in knee flexion and extension.

b. What ligaments guide the femoral condyles in anterior and posterior gliding.

c. Using the Rule of Three, describe the spinning taking place in the knee during terminal extension in the open and closed kinematic chain situations. What function does this spinning accomplish?

10. What is considered to be full range of motion at the knee? Make sure you give the figures for all of the motions in the knee.

11. Explain the screw-home mechanism, including its kinesiological usefulness and the muscle responsible for the unlocking of the knee.

12. In what position of the knee are the medial and lateral collateral ligaments most lax? Taut?

13. In what position of the knee is the anterior cruciate ligament on greatest tension? In what position of the knee is the posterior cruciate ligament on greatest tension?

14. Considering the answers to the ligament tension and screw-home mechanism questions above, what is the close-packed position of the knee? Since rotation of the tibia on the femur is impossible in the close-packed position, you can use this movement to verify your answer.

15. What intrajoint structures occupy sufficient space to keep the joint ligaments taut in extension?

16. Which meniscus is most firmly attached to the tibia and joint capsule?

17. Describe the movement of the medial and lateral menisci as the knee:
   a. Extends

   b. Flexes

18. What forces create the meniscal movements described in item 17?

19. Describe the physiological and accessory movements of the patella.

20. Explain (and diagram on Figure 5-6) patellar tracking and the mechanisms by which it is controlled. In your discussion and diagram, include at least:

   a. Vectors representing muscle forces acting on the patella during active extension of the tibia at the knee and the resultant of those forces
   b. Connective tissue support of the patella
   c. Bony configuration of the patellofemoral joint

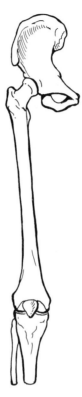

FIGURE 5–6

*21. For this activity, you will need a subject in shorts. Have the subject sit on the edge of a treatment table with feet dangling over the side. Passively extend the right tibia at the knee so that the knee is straight. Ask the subject to remain relaxed so that there is no active tension in the right quadriceps as you gradually flex the knee. As you flex the knee, passively move the patella medially and laterally at various points in the range of motion.

   a. At what angle of knee flexion are you no longer able to move the patella?

   b. What is the relationship or orientation of the patellar and femoral articular surfaces at that angle?

c. What will be the primary effect on the patellofemoral joint of an isometric contraction of the quadriceps at that angle?

d. Passively extend the knee fully and ask for another isometric quadriceps contraction. What is the primary effect on the patellofemoral joint of the isometric contraction in this position?

e. State a principle concerning the effect on the patellofemoral joint of quadriceps contraction at various knee-joint angles.

*22. Measure the Q angle on four subjects. Be sure that there is a mix of male and female subjects.

a. What landmarks did you use to obtain the measurement?

b. How will an increase in this angle affect patellar tracking?

23. What bursae of the knee are most likely compressed between the floor and the knee when you are kneeling?

MYOLOGY OF THE KNEE

Use the following muscle sheets to aid in learning the origins, insertions, and innervations of the knee muscles. For each of the muscles named, draw in the muscle on the sketch provided and complete the indicated information on the outline.

O: Origin of muscle
I: Insertion of muscle
N: Innervation (both peripheral nerve and spinal level)
R: Relationship of muscle to axis of motion
A: Action of muscle

24. Quadriceps femoris

    Rectus femoris (see description in Chapter 4)

    Vastus intermedius

    O: Anterior and lateral surfaces of proximal femoral shaft

    I:

    N: Femoral n. (L-2, L-3, L-4)

    R: Fibers run straight (superior and inferior) from O to I; anterior to axis for flexion and extension

    A: Extension of the tibia at the knee

    Vastus medialis

    O: Distal portion of intertrochanteric line of femur; medial lip of linea aspera; proximal part of medial supracondylar ridge

    I:

    N: Femoral n. (L-2, L-3, L-4)

    R:

    A: Extension of the tibia at the knee

    Vastus lateralis

    O:

    I: Lateral border of patella and then to the tibial tuberosity via the patellar ligament

    N: Femoral n. (L-2, L-3, L-4)

    R:

    A: Extension of the tibia at the knee

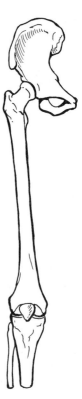

FIGURE 5–6

25. Popliteus

    O:

    I:

    N: Tibial n. (L-4, L-5, S-1)

    R: Fibers run obliquely and inferiorly from O to I; posterior and medial to axis for rotation of tibia at the knee; posterior and lateral to axis for rotation of femur at the knee

    A:

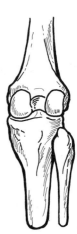

FIGURE 5–7

26. Plantaris

   O:
   I: Tendocalcaneus
   N:
   R: Fibers run superior and inferior from O to I, in the form of a long, slender tendon; posterior to axes for ankle dorsiflexion and plantarflexion, and for knee flexion and extension
   A: Weak plantarflexion of foot at the ankle; flexion of tibia at the knee

27. Gastrocnemius

   O:
   I: Tendocalcaneus; posterior surface of calcaneus
   N: Tibial n. (S-1, S-2)
   R:
   A: Plantar flexion of the foot at the ankle and flexion of the tibia at the knee

28. Hamstrings (see Chapter 4 for their description)

29. List all the one-joint muscles crossing the knee.

30. List the muscles crossing posterior to the knee joint.

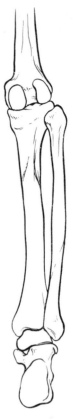

FIGURE 5–8

APPLICATIONS

*31. Passively flex a subject's knee to 90° and perform passive medial rotation of the tibia at the knee to the end range. The end feel will be firm, indicating that the motion is restricted by ligament. Now, passively laterally rotate the tibia. You should find a similar end-feel at the limit of the range of motion. What ligaments are restricting the motion in each case? Note: If you have difficulty figuring out the answer to this question from reading and discussion, try the movements on a cadaver in gross anatomy laboratory, once the knee is dissected and the ligaments can be viewed.

*32. With your subject sitting, muscle-test the quadriceps with the subject leaning forward and then leaning back. What difference in muscle strength did you find? Explain the difference.

*33. Determine a position for muscle-testing the quadriceps group that allows the greatest tension to be developed by the entire muscle group through the greatest range of motion. Perform the test and compare your results with the standard position for muscle-testing the quadriceps. Was there a difference in strength in the two positions? If there was, explain why.

*34. Muscle-test the hamstrings with the ankle plantarflexed and then with the ankle dorsiflexed. Did you find a difference in strength in the two positions? Explain your results.

*35. Perform a reasonable test of hamstring strength that requires the muscle to work against gravity through the full range of motion. Be sure to allow the muscle to develop maximum tension through maximum range of motion.

*36. Examine the effect on the lumbar spine (in a standing subject) of moving the knees from a normal to a recurvatum position.

*37. Examine the effect on the lumbar spine (in a standing subject) of moving the knees from a normal to a mildly flexed position.

*38. Perform a break test for knee extension with the subject's knee fully extended and then with it flexed 5°. In which position was it easier to break the contraction? Why?

*39. These activities are best done by an individual with normally stable knees.
   a. From an erect standing position, cross the left lower limb in front of the right and place it on the ground, turning to the right while the right foot remains stationary. (The right lower limb will be twisted.)
      What position does the right femur assume in relation to the tibia?

      What knee ligaments are most stressed in this position?

   b. In a normal standing position, what knee ligaments would be most stressed by a sudden valgus stress?

40. Explain the biomechanical and functional implications of a patellectomy. Be sure to include moment arms in your discussion.

41. What muscle group would you strengthen to provide dynamic stability to substitute for the loss of stability of a torn anterior cruciate ligament? Explain your choice.

*42. Explain why a positive Apley's compression test with lateral rotation of the tibia on the femur is indicative of a tear in the posterior horn of the medial meniscus. A positive test means that the patient complains of pain during the maneuver.

43. As you move from squatting to standing, the femur extends at the knee, producing a rolling of the femoral condyles on the tibial plateau. Explain the intrajoint mechanics that prevent crushing of the menisci and anterior dislocation of the femur off the tibia during this movement.

ANSWERS TO KNEE

1. Lateral epicondyle, femur*
   Lateral condyle, femur*
   Medial epicondyle, femur*
   Medial condyle, femur*
   Adductor tubercle*
   Patellar surface of femur
   Apex of patella*
   Base of patella*
   Patellar facet for lateral femoral condyle
   Patellar facet for medial femoral condyle
   Medial condyle of tibia
   Tubercles of intercondylar eminence
   Lateral condyle of tibia
   Head of fibula*
   Tibial tuberosity*

2. The posterior surface of the patella is multifaceted with a central longitudinal ridge covered with articular cartilage. The central ridge separates the two main articular surfaces, the medial and lateral.

3. The medial condyle projects more distally than the lateral, helping to produce the normal valgus in the knee.

4. Check your anatomy text for confirmation of your drawing. In addition to the area of attachment to the coronary ligaments, shade the areas where the transverse ligament joins the two menisci, where the semimembranosus muscle and the medial collateral ligament are attached to the medial meniscus, and where the meniscofemoral ligament and popliteus muscle are attached to the lateral meniscus.

5. Check your text and have a faculty member confirm your information.

*6. Have a faculty member confirm your palpations. Deduction of the stress position for each ligament can be made from the structure and function of the ligament. For instance, since the medial collateral ligament resists a valgus stress of the knee and since it is lax in some flexion of the knee, it can be palpated by first relaxing it then placing the knee on a valgus stress. Palpating the medial joint line during the valgus maneuver will locate the ligament as it changes from lax to taut. Repeat the problem-solving process for determining the position for palpating the lateral collateral ligament.

7. The joint surfaces within the articular capsule of the knee are the patellar and complementary femoral surface of the patellofemoral joint, the femoral condyles, and the tibial plateau. The menisci are also within the capsule. The cruciate ligaments reside outside the synovial cavity of the articular capsule, but have independent synovial covering.

8. The knee is not a true hinge joint because it has two degrees of freedom, rotation as well as flexion and extension.

9. a. Gliding maintains the larger joint surface of the femur in contact with the tibia, gliding it forward during flexion of the femur on the tibia, and gliding it back during extension of the femur on the tibia.
   b. The anterior cruciate controls backward roll of the femoral condyles on the tibial plateau during flexion of the femur at the knee. This guides the anterior glide of the femoral condyles on the tibial plateau during flexion of the femur at the knee. The posterior cruciate does the opposite.
   c. In the open kinematic chain, the tibia laterally rotates at the knee at terminal extension. In the closed chain, the femur medially rotates at the knee. This stabilizes the knee when it is in full extension.

10. Full range of motion at the knee is 135° of active flexion of the tibia at the knee and 40° to 80° of passive rotation of tibia at the knee (depending on author) with the knee at 90° of flexion. About 20° of rotation of the tibia at the knee occur at terminal extension. The figures are the same for the reverse actions.

11. Medial rotation of the femur at the knee (closed kinematic chain), or lateral rotation of the tibia at the knee (open kinematic chain) accomplishes the screw-home mechanism and seats the intercondylar tubercles of the tibia into the intercondylar notch of the femur. It also brings the collateral and cruciate ligaments into their tightest position and seats the femoral condyles tightly into the menisci.

    The locked-knee position allows standing without active contraction of the antigravity knee muscles. The muscle that unlocks the knee is the popliteus.

12. The medial and lateral collateral ligaments are most lax at 90° of flexion and taut at full extension. They are, of course, also relatively lax between full extension and 90° of flexion, although some portion of the medial collateral ligament is taut throughout the range of flexion and extension.

13. Both cruciates are taut in extension, with the anterior cruciate relatively more so than the posterior. Some fibers of the anterior cruciate are taut throughout the range of motion of flexion and extension. The posterior portion of the posterior cruciate is taut in full extension, whereas the anterior portion is taut in flexion.

14. Full extension is the close-packed position of the knee. The bones are fully congruent and the greatest number of stabilizing ligaments are at their tightest in this position. No rotation is possible in the extended position.

15. The menisci and articular cartilage occupy space and maintain the tension on the ligaments. Loss of these space-occupying tissues causes approximation of the joint surfaces and laxity in the ligaments.

16. The medial meniscus is attached to the medial collateral ligament and the medial capsule. It is more firmly attached to the tibial plateau than the lateral meniscus.

17. a. The menisci slide anteriorly as the knee extends. The lateral meniscus moves further than the medial.
    b. They move posteriorly during flexion.

18. Anterior movement is accomplished by pull from the meniscopatellar ligaments and by the fact that the femoral condyles are rolling anteriorly against the ridges of the menisci. During flexion, they move posteriorly in response to the rolling of the femoral condyles, plus the semimembranosus pulls the medial meniscus posteriorly and the popliteus pulls the lateral meniscus posteriorly by active contraction.

19. The patella is anchored firmly to the tibia by the patellar ligament, so its superior-inferior movement is dependent on movement of the tibia. As the tibia moves into flexion at the knee, it pulls the patella inferiorly in relation to the femur. As the quadriceps pull the tibia into extension at the knee, the patella moves superiorly on the femur.

    In the extended but relaxed position, the patella can be passively moved in medial-lateral and superior-inferior directions.

20. The patella tracks superiorly and inferiorly in the intercondylar groove. Whether it tracks in midline, medially, or laterally depends on the relative forces of the medial and lateral vasti and the patellar retinaculum. The medial and lateral lips of the intercondylar groove of the femur also tend to guide the movement of the patella. If there is asymmetry in the controlling forces, then it will track to the side with the stronger influence.

*21. a. The angle of flexion when the patella becomes fixed medially and laterally varies according to individuals.

    b. The patellar articular surfaces are well down the femoral articular surfaces and seated in the interarticular groove. The patella is approaching the distal end of the femur and a position more perpendicular than parallel to the shaft of the femur.

    c. The primary effect will be compression of the patellofemoral joint surfaces.

    d. In full extension, the patella is parallel to the shaft of the femur, and contraction of the quadriceps will produce sliding of the patella in the articular groove of the femur, rather than compression against the femur.

    e. With greater flexion of the knee joint, contraction of the quadriceps causes greater compression in the patellofemoral joint. More recent research indicates that the angle of greatest patellofemoral compression may vary depending on whether the knee is in an open or closed kinematic chain.

*22. The normal Q angle varies from 10° to 20°; female subjects normally show a larger angle.

    a. ASIS, midpatella, tibial tuberosity

    b. An increase in the angle will create a bowstring effect since the patella is tethered between the superiorly pulling quadriceps and the inferiorly pulling patellar ligament. The increased Q angle causes greater lateral force on the patella, producing greater pressure on the lateral lip of the articular groove of the femur as well as on the lateral articular surface of the patella.

23. The bursae are the prepatellar and infrapatellar.

24. Quadriceps femoris

    a. Rectus femoris (see description in Chapter 4)

    b. Vastus intermedius

        O: Anterior and lateral surfaces of proximal femoral shaft
        I: Base of patella and then to the tibial tuberosity via the patellar ligament
        N: Femoral n. (L-2, L-3, L-4)
        R: Fibers run straight (superior and inferior) from O to I; anterior to axis for flexion and extension
        A: Extension of the tibia at the knee

    c. Vastus medialis

        O: Distal portion of intertrochanteric line; medial lip of linea aspera; proximal part of medial supracondylar ridge
        I: Medial border of patella and then to the tibial tuberosity via the patellar ligament
        N: Femoral n. (L-2, L-3, L-4)
        R: Fibers run straight (superior and inferior) from O to I; anterior to axis for flexion and extension (most medial of quadriceps and therefore pulls the patella medially)
        A: Extension of the tibia at the knee

    d. Vastus lateralis

        O: Anterior portion of greater trochanter; proximal portion of intertrochanteric line; proximal half of lateral lip of linea aspera
        I: Lateral border of patella and then to the tibial tuberosity via the patellar ligament
        N: Femoral n. (L-2, L-3, L-4)
        R: Fibers run straight (superior and inferior) from O to I; anterior to axis for flexion and extension (most lateral of the quadriceps and therefore pulls the patella laterally)
        A: Extension of the tibia at the knee

25. Popliteus

    O: Posterior surface of lateral epicondyle of femur
    I: Posterior surface of medial proximal tibia
    N: Tibial n. (L-4, L-5, S-1)
    R: Fibers run obliquely and inferiorly from O to I; posterior and medial to axis for rotation of tibia at the knee; posterior and lateral to axis for rotation of femur at the knee
    A: Medial rotation of tibia at the knee (open kinematic chain); lateral rotation of the femur at the knee (closed kinematic chain)

26. Plantaris

   O: Posterior surface of lateral epicondyle of femur
   I: Tendocalcaneus
   N: Tibial n. (L-5, S-1)
   R: Fibers run superior and inferior from O to I, in the form of a long, slender tendon; posterior to axes for ankle dorsiflexion and plantarflexion, and for knee flexion and extension
   A: Weak plantarflexion of foot at the ankle; flexion of tibia at the knee

27. Gastrocnemius

   O: Posterior surface of medial and lateral epicondyles of femur
   I: Tendocalcaneus; posterior surface of calcaneus
   N: Tibial n. (S-1, S-2)
   R: From each origin to midline of muscle to form two heads; posterior to axis for knee flexion and extension; posterior to axis for ankle plantarflexion and dorsiflexion
   A: Plantar flexion of the foot at the ankle; flexion of the tibia at the knee

28. Hamstrings (see Chapter 4)

29. The one-joint muscles crossing the knee are the

   Biceps short head
   Popliteus
   Vastus lateralis
   Vastus intermedius
   Vastus medialis

30. The muscles crossing posterior to the knee are the

   Hamstrings
   Popliteus
   Gastrocnemius
   Plantaris

*31. This activity reinforces the sensation of a ligamentous end-feel and can lead into the mechanics of knee ligament injuries. The firm end-feel at the end-range of medial rotation of the tibia on the femur is the result of tightening of the anterior and posterior cruciate ligaments; in lateral rotation, it is of the medial and lateral collateral ligaments.

*32. This activity demonstrates a functional relevance of active insufficiency and body position during exercise or muscle-testing. It also can lead to discussion of the relative contribution of the rectus femoris to the force of the quadriceps and the effect of hip position on that force.

*33. There are several possible solutions to this problem. However, each must satisfy the criterion of preventing active insufficiency in the rectus as the knee approaches full extension.

*34. This is another length-tension relationship problem, demonstrating how a muscle with primary function at the ankle (gastrocnemius) can affect the force of flexion of the tibia at the knee. The learners will most likely find that knee flexion is stronger with the ankle dorsiflexed than with it plantarflexed. This can lead to the rationalization of the hamstring muscle-testing position with the ankle plantarflexed.

*35. Again, there are many possible solutions, but they must all position the limb so that flexion of the tibia is never assisted by gravity and must allow hip motion to compensate for the hamstring muscle shortening over the knee. An example could be to position the subject in a standing position and have her simultaneously flex her hip and knee.

*36. Genu recurvatum produces a compensatory increase in lumbar lordosis.

*37. Standing with knee flexion produces a compensatory decrease in lumbar lordosis.

*38. The learners should find it easier to break the isometric contraction with the knee slightly flexed because the fully extended knee is locked and has ligamentous stability, while the partially flexed knee relies mainly on muscle strength to maintain the position.

*39. a. Lateral rotation; cruciates
   b. Medial collateral; anterior cruciate

40. Removal of the patella removes the pulley effect for the quadriceps over the knee, thus bringing the line of pull of the muscle closer to the axis of motion. This change in line of pull of the quadriceps decreases the moment arm of the muscle force, thus diminishing the effective strength of the muscle. Patellectomy functionally weakens the quadriceps.

41. The hamstrings, because of their line of pull, put a posterior translatory force on the tibia, pulling it posteriorly on the femur as well as rotating the tibia into flexion.

42. The meniscus is compressed as the tibia is pressed downward onto the condyle of the femur. Lateral rotation of the tibia asymmetrically stresses the posterior horn of the medial meniscus.

43. The condyles of the femur glide posteriorly as the knee extends because of the tethering provided by the posterior cruciate ligament. This keeps the articular surfaces in contact and the femur on the tibia. The rolling of the femoral condyles and the pull of the meniscopatellar ligaments bring the menisci forward, avoiding their compression between the condyles and the tibial plateau.

6 FOOT AND ANKLE

OSTEOLOGY OF THE FOOT AND ANKLE

The Foot

1. On Figures 6-1 to 6-3, identify and label the bones listed below. Familiarize yourself with these bones and landmarks by identifying them in text drawings and on a skeleton.

Phalanges	Tuberosity of cuboid
Metatarsals	Talus (head and neck)
Tubercles of metatarsals	Calcaneus
Tuberosity of fifth metatarsal	Sustentaculum tali
Cuneiforms	Peroneal tubercle of calcaneus
Cuboid	Navicular tubercle

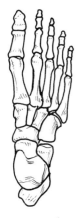

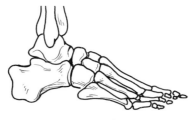

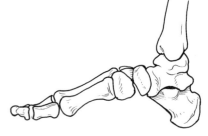

FIGURE 6–1   **FIGURE 6–2**   **FIGURE 6–3**

2. What is the function of the sustentaculum tali of the calcaneus?

3. What is the function of the navicular tuberosity?

The Ankle

*4. Familiarize yourself with the structures listed below by identifying them on the skeleton and then palpating them on yourself and a classmate.

Medial malleolus
Lateral malleolus
Distal portion of shaft of tibia
Distal portion of shaft of fibula
Joint line of talocrural joint

5. What is the function of the sulcus tali of the talus?

6. Define tibial torsion. How does normal tibial torsion affect the foot in stance? What is the normal amount of tibial torsion evident during stance?

7. Define external or lateral and internal or medial tibial torsion.

ARTHROLOGY OF THE FOOT AND ANKLE

8. Complete the outline below:

Superior tibiofibular joint
Type of joint

Bones involved

Movement(s) permitted

Inferior tibiofibular joint
Type of joint

Bones involved

Movement(s) permitted

Talocrural joint
   Type of joint

   Bones involved

   Movement(s) permitted

Subtalar (talocalcaneal) joint
   Type of joint

   Bones involved

   Movement(s) permitted

Talocalcaneonavicular joint
   Type of joint

   Bones involved

   Movement(s) permitted

Calcaneocuboid joint
   Type of joint

   Bones involved

   Movement(s) permitted

Talonavicular joint
   Type of joint

   Bones involved

   Movement(s) permitted

Transverse tarsal joint
   Type of joint

   Bones involved

   Movement(s) permitted

Tarsometatarsal joints
   Type of joint

   Bones involved

   Movement(s) permitted

Metatarsophalangeal joints
   Type of joint

   Bones involved

   Movement(s) permitted

Interphalangeal joints
   Type of joint

Bones involved

Movement(s) permitted

*9. With your laboratory partner sitting on a treatment table with his legs extended on the table, hold the distal end of his tibia firmly. With your other hand, try to move the distal end of the fibula posteriorly (down toward the table). What, if any, motion do you feel? What limits motion at the inferior tibiofibular joint?

10. Why is the talocrural joint referred to as a mortise-and-tenon joint?

11. In view of the shape of the articular surface of the talus, what motion is required of the mortise during dorsi-flexion?

*12. Passively take your partner's foot into full pronation and full supination. In which direction were you able to obtain more motion? What is the relationship of your finding to the asymmetry between the medial and lateral malleoli?

13. Define the following terms as they apply to movements of the foot and ankle. Go to several sources for your definitions. You will probably note that different sources use the same terms to mean different motions. It will be important for you to be aware of all of the definitions so that you can communicate accurately about ankle motions.

Dorsiflexion:

Plantarflexion:

Inversion:

Eversion:

Pronation:

Supination:

Abduction:

Adduction:

14. Which foot and ankle joints are primarily responsible for supination (making the soles of the feet face each other) and pronation (making the soles of the feet face away from each other)? In other words, if you wanted to surgically eliminate these motions, what joints would you need to fuse?

*15. Sit with your right shoe and sock off and your right ankle crossed over your left thigh, right foot unsupported. Completely relax your right foot and move your calcaneus up and down by pushing up under the lateral side with your fingers and letting it flop back down. Do this repeatedly so that you can see the motion between the calcaneus and the talus. The arc ascribed by the foot approximates the arc of motion of the calcaneus.

    a. Describe the arc that you see. Note that it crosses three planes of motion.

    b. Give the component open-chain subtalar motions for:
    Pronation

    Supination

*16. Reverse action in the subtalar joint is a wondrous thing to understand. To help, we will start with superimposed fists, ulnar side of your left fist above and touching the radial side of your right fist; MP joint knuckles of both hands vertically aligned. The right fist is the calcaneus and the left is the talus of the left foot.

    a. Perform open-chain pronation of the joint. Note: Consult your answer to item 15b for the components of calcaneal motion contained in open-chain pronation of the subtalar joint and simulate them with your right fist. Remember the relative position of your MP joint knuckles once you have achieved the position.

    b. Perform the reverse action of subtalar pronation with the talus moving and the calcaneus holding still, i.e., closed-chain pronation. Your knuckles should end up in the same relative position as they did in open-chain pronation.

    c. Since the tibia is intimately tied to the talus, it will move when the talus moves. What motion will occur in the left tibia during closed-chain pronation of the left subtalar joint?

17. In which position is the transverse tarsal joint close-packed?

18. In which position is the transverse tarsal joint open-packed?

19. Which of the tarsometatarsal joints share a joint capsule?

20. What is the function of the metatarsophalangeal joint in the weight-bearing foot?

21. What is the function of the interphalangeal joints of the toes in the weight-bearing foot?

22. What is the primary function of the ligaments of the ankle-foot complex? Why do we attend to these ligaments in more detail than with some other joints?

23. a. What is the specific function of the anterior tibiofibular, posterior tibiofibular, and crural interosseous tibiofibular ligaments?

   b. Draw the crural interosseous tibiofibular ligament on Figure 6-4.

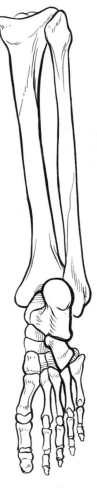

FIGURE 6–4

   c. Draw and label the anterior tibiofibular and posterior tibiofibular ligaments on Figure 6-2.

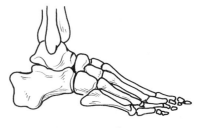

FIGURE 6–2

*24. a. What is the specific function of the anterior talofibular, posterior talofibular, calcaneofibular, long plantar, and short plantar ligaments?

    b. Draw and label each ligament on Figures 6–2 and 6-3 in item 1.
    c. Passively stress each of the ligaments.
    d. Palpate each of the ligaments that are palpable.

25. In an inversion-plantarflexion injury, which ligaments are most likely to be injured?

26. Which of the lateral ligaments is the weakest?

*27. a. What is the function of the deltoid ligament and the spring ligament?

    b. Draw the four parts of the deltoid ligament and the spring ligament on Figure 6-3. Label the parts of the deltoid ligament.

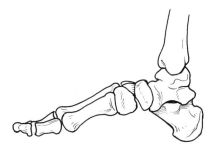

FIGURE 6–3

    c. Stress the deltoid and spring ligaments.
    d. Palpate the deltoid ligament.
    e. Palpate the calcaneal attachment of the spring ligament.

28. a. High stress in what position could cause disruption of the deltoid ligament?

   b. Is disruption of this ligament likely?

   c. Why or why not?

29. What are the attachments and function of the deep transverse metatarsal ligament?

ARCHES OF THE FOOT

30. Complete the following outline:

   Medial longitudinal arch
      Bones involved:

      Major support:

   Lateral longitudinal arch
      Bones involved:

      Major support:

   Transverse arch
      Bones involved:

      Major support:

31. On Figure 6-5, draw in the plantar fascia with its major attachments. What is the effect of extension of the MP joints on tension of the plantar fascia?

*32. Examine the medial longitudinal arch of three subjects. To do that, draw a line from the distal portion of the medial malleolus to the head of the first metatarsal. Observe where the navicular tubercle falls in relation to that line (above, below, or on it). What anatomical structures, in addition to what you listed in item 30, are responsible for maintaining this arch? Was there much variation in the results from one subject to the next?

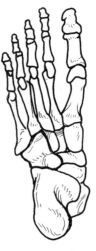

FIGURE 6–5

MYOLOGY OF THE FOOT AND ANKLE

Use the following muscle sheets to aid in learning the origins, insertions, and innervations of the foot muscles. For each muscle named, draw in the muscle on the sketch and complete the indicated information on the outline. The following abbreviations apply throughout the muscle sheets:

O: Origin of muscle
 I: Insertion of muscle
N: Innervation (both spinal level and peripheral nerve)
R: Relationship of muscle to axis of motion
A: Action of muscle

33. Tibialis posterior

O: Medial surface of proximal two thirds of fibula; interosseous membrane; posterolateral surface of tibia

 I: Tuberosity of navicular; plantar surfaces of sustentaculum of calcaneus; three cuneiforms; cuboid; bases of second, third, and fourth metatarsals (does not attach to talus posteriorly or to first and fifth metatarsal anteriorly)

N: Tibial n. (L-5, S-1)

R: Courses straight and slightly anteriorly; winds around posterior surface of medial malleolus; enters the sole of the foot; winds around talus and then divides into its numerous insertions; medial to axis for inversion and eversion

A:

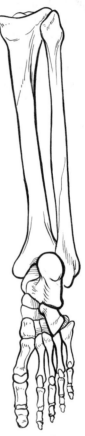

FIGURE 6–4

34. Peroneus longus

   O: Superior two thirds of lateral surface of fibula

   I: Lateral aspect of base of first metatarsal and medial cuneiform

   N: Superficial peroneal n. (L-4, L-5, S-1)

   R: Tendon courses inferiorly and winds around posterior aspect of lateral malleolus; continues in a groove on plantar surface of cuboid; crosses plantar surface of foot to reach insertion; lateral to axis for inversion and eversion; slightly posterior to axis for dorsiflexion and plantarflexion

   A:

35. Peroneus brevis

   O:

   I:

   N:

   R:

   A:

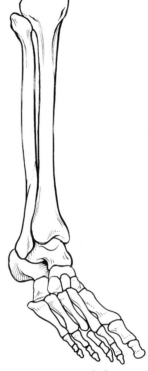

FIGURE 6–6

36. Tibialis anterior

   O:

   I:

   N:

   R:

   A:

37. Extensor digitorum longus

   O:

   I:

   N:

   R:

   A:

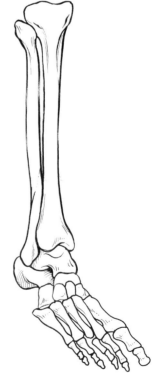

FIGURE 6–6

38. Extensor digitorum brevis

    O:
    I:
    N:
    R:
    A:

39. Extensor hallucis longus

    O:
    I:
    N:
    R:
    A:

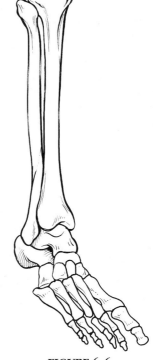

FIGURE 6–6

40. Gastrocnemius

    O:
    I:
    N:
    R:
    A:

41. Soleus

    O:
    I:
    N:
    R:
    A:

42. Plantaris

    O:
    I:
    N:
    R:
    A:

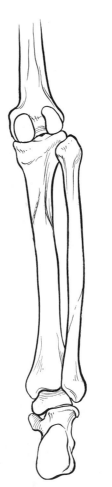
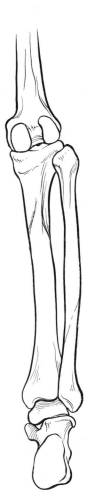

FIGURE 6–7

43. Flexor digitorum brevis

   O: Calcaneus
    I: Middle phalanges of lateral four toes
   N: Medial plantar n. (L-4, L-5)
   R:
   A:

44. Abductor hallucis

   O:
    I:
   N:
   R:
   A:

45. Flexor hallucis longus

   O: Lower two thirds of posterior fibula
    I: Base of distal phalanx of great toe
   N: Tibial n. (L-5, S-1, S-2)
   R: Plantar to axis for flexion and extension; posterior
       to axis for dorsiflexion and plantarflexion
   A:

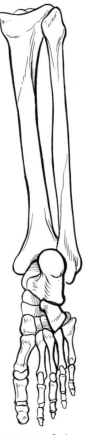

FIGURE 6–4

46. Flexor digitorum longus

   O:
    I:
   N:
   R:
   A:

47. Peroneus longus tendon (see item 34)

48. Tibialis posterior tendon (see item 33)

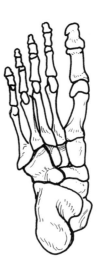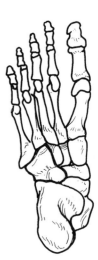

FIGURE 6–5

APPLICATIONS

*49. Test the strength of the gastrocnemius with the knee fully flexed and with the knee extended. Note the difference in strength of contraction of the gastrocnemius with the knee flexed versus with the knee extended. What principle does this illustrate? What are the implications of this for manual muscle-testing?

*50. Place your partner's limb in the most effective position to lengthen (stretch) the gastrocnemius muscle. Explain.

*51. Demonstrate an isolated contraction of each of the muscles listed below. What instructions would be helpful to a patient to accomplish these isolated contractions? Be able to palpate each tendon.

    a. Tibialis anterior
    b. Extensor hallucis longus
    c. Extensor digitorum longus

52. Explain why strengthening the peroneus longus and brevis is important following an inversion sprain of the ankle.

*53. In small groups, work with an articulated skeleton of the foot and ankle. Complete and discuss the following motions.

    a. In an open kinematic chain, laterally rotate the tibia on the femur. In what position does this place the foot? How does lateral rotation of the tibia reorient the axis of the ankle joint?

    b. In an open kinematic chain, medially rotate the tibia on the femur. In what position does this place the foot? How does medial rotation of the tibia reorient the axis of the ankle joint?

    c. In a closed kinematic chain, laterally rotate the tibia on the femur but keep the foot flat on the floor. In what position does this place the foot? What other joints of the foot are affected by closed-chain lateral rotation of the tibia?

    d. In a closed kinematic chain, medially rotate the tibia on the femur but keep the foot flat on the floor. In what position does this place the foot? What other joints of the foot are affected by closed-chain medial rotation of the tibia?

*54. Now repeat the above tibial motions with a subject who is wearing shorts and is barefoot. Note the relationship between the closed-chain and open-chain tibial rotation and the movement of the foot.

*55. Stand with your leg and foot exposed, foot flat on the ground and knee slightly bent to avoid the screw-home-locking mechanism limiting movement of the tibia at the knee. Pronate your right foot by depressing the medial longitudinal arch toward the floor.

    a. What movement occurs in the tibia as the foot pronates?

    b. What posture tends to occur at the knee with closed-chain foot pronation?

*56. What other major joint(s) of the body would be affected by pathological pronation of the foot in stance? How would they be affected? Demonstrate your explanation with an articulated skeleton of a knee, foot, and ankle.

*57. On a laboratory partner, palpate the following structures:

First metatarsocuneiform joint	Lateral malleolus
Navicular tubercle	Metatarsal heads
Medial malleolus	Dorsal pedal pulse
Fifth metatarsal bone	Tibialis posterior tendon to insertion
Fifth metatarsophalangeal joint	Peroneus brevis tendon to insertion
Calcaneus	Peroneus tertius tendon
Sustentaculum tali	Tibialis anterior tendon
Peroneal tubercle	Extensor hallucis longus tendon

*58. On your partner, put a dot over the base of the fifth metatarsal and another dot over the head of the fifth metatarsal. Have your partner sit on a treatment table with the knee flexed and the foot over the edge. Position the foot so that the sole of the foot is parallel to the floor. Are the two dots in a line parallel to the floor? What are the implications of this for goniometry of the ankle?

*59. Measure at least five classmates for tibial torsion (amount of toe-out with the tibia facing directly forward); you can measure this with a goniometer. What variation among individuals did you find? Were any of these individuals considered abnormal?

*60. Measure ankle dorsiflexion with the knee extended, then with the knee flexed. Did you find a difference in measurement between the two positions? If you did, explain why you did.

ANSWERS TO FOOT AND ANKLE

1. Check your text and confirm your information with a faculty member.

2. The shelflike projection of the calcaneus known as the sustentaculum tali articulates with and supports the talus and serves as attachment for the spring ligament.

3. Attachment for the tibialis posterior.

*4. Check with your text and confirm your information with a faculty member.

5. The deep groove of the talus, the sulcus tali, serves as the attachment for the interosseous ligament between the talus and calcaneus.

6. The torsion or twisting of the distal tibia laterally as compared to the proximal portion is called tibial torsion. This produces a toe-out position of the foot in relation to the leg of 20° to 30°.

7. External or lateral tibial torsion is a pathological increase in tibial torsion. Internal or medial tibial torsion is the pathological decrease in tibial torsion.

8. Superior tibiofibular joint

   Type of joint: plane, synovial joint
   Bones involved: fibula and tibia
   Movements permitted: slight superior and inferior gliding of the fibula and fibular rotation

   Inferior tibiofibular joint
   Type of joint: syndesmosis
   Bones involved: tibia and fibula
   Movements permitted: slight separation and gliding

   Talocrural joint
   Type of joint: hinge, synovial joint
   Bones involved: talus, tibia, and fibula
   Movements permitted: dorsiflexion and plantarflexion

   Subtalar (talocalcaneal) joint
   Type of joint: plane, synovial joint
   Bones involved: talus and calcaneus
   Movements permitted: supination and pronation

   Talocalcaneonavicular joint
   Type of joint: plane, synovial joint
   Bones involved: talus, navicular, and calcaneus
   Movements permitted: supination and pronation

   Calcaneocuboid joint
   Type of joint: plane, synovial joint
   Bones involved: calcaneus and cuboid
   Movements permitted: supination and pronation

   Talonavicular joint
   Type of joint: plane, synovial joint
   Bones involved: talus and navicular
   Movements permitted: supination and pronation

   Transverse tarsal joint
   Type of joint: compound, plane, synovial joint
   Bones involved: talus and navicular; calcaneus and cuboid
   Movements permitted: supination and pronation

Tarsometatarsal joints
  Type of joint: plane, synovial joint
  Bones involved: distal tarsal row and metatarsals
  Movements permitted: supination and pronation opposite to the closed chain motion of the subtalar and transverse tarsal joints to keep the forefoot in contact with the ground

Metatarsophalangeal joints
  Type of joint: condyloid, synovial joint
  Bones involved: metatarsals and phalanges
  Movements permitted: extension, flexion, abduction, and adduction

Interphalangeal joints
  Type of joint: hinge, synovial joint
  Bones involved: phalanges
  Movements permitted: flexion and extension

*9. Some motion is available in this direction. It is limited by fibroadipose tissue and interosseous ligament.

10. The tibia and fibula form an almost-rectangular concave articular surface for the almost-rectangular convex talar head to articulate with. This resembles a mortise-and-tenon joint in carpentry.

11. The trochlea rotates posteriorly in the ankle mortise with dorsiflexion. The malleoli tend to separate because the superior articular surface of the talus is wider anteriorly than posteriorly.

*12. You were probably able to obtain more supination than pronation. The more distal position of the lateral malleolus serves to limit the motion of the ankle in pronation. Functionally, this increases the stability of the ankle.

13. Use your texts to confirm your answers.

14. Pronation is a combination of abduction, eversion, and dorsiflexion of the foot and ankle. Supination is a combination of adduction, inversion, and plantarflexion of the foot and ankle. The talocalcaneal, talonavicular, and calcaneocuboid joints are primarily responsible for supination and pronation. To eliminate the motions, all three joints would have to be fused. This procedure is called a triple arthrodesis.

15. a. You should see an arc that includes dorsiflexion/plantarflexion; inversion/eversion, and adduction/abduction of the foot.
    b. In open-chain subtalar motion, the calcaneus is moving on the talus. Supination includes plantarflexion, adduction, and inversion of the calcaneus on the talus. Pronation includes dorsiflexion, abduction, and eversion of the calcaneus on the talus.

*16. a. Simulating the triplanar movement of the calcaneus is not easy and may need some verification from a colleague as you work it out.
    b. You will quickly realize that the left hand must move in exactly the opposite attitudes to those the right performed in part a. The same is true for talar movement on the calcaneus during pronation of the foot while in contact with the floor, and the calcaneus is immobile for plantar and dorsiflexion.
    c. The important aspect of this exercise is what happens when talar motion is translated to the tibia and the tibia moves or changes position. In the case of closed-chain subtalar pronation, the talus adducts (medially rotates), so the tibia will medially rotate. Can you see this from the movement of your hands? Remember that your hands represent the talus and calcaneus of the *left* foot. This phenomenon will be addressed again in the applications section.

17. The transverse tarsal joint is close-packed in supination.

18. The transverse tarsal joint is open-packed in pronation.

19. The second and third tarsometatarsal joints share a joint capsule. The fourth and fifth tarsometatarsal joints share a joint capsule. Gliding or sliding motions occur at these joints.

20. The metatarsophalangeal joints allow the rigid supinated foot to pass over the weight-bearing toes.

*21. The interphalangeal joints help maintain stability by pressing into the ground in static posture and during ambulation as needed. During gait, weight is shifted by the toes to the opposite foot.

22. Static stabilization. The ankle ligaments are commonly injured; therefore, their position and function need to be well understood.

23. a. Maintaining a stable mortise.
    b and c. Check your text to confirm your information.

*24. a. The anterior talofibular, posterior talofibular, and calcaneofibular ligaments limit distraction of the talus from the fibula (this might occur in severe inversion). The long and short plantar ligaments help to maintain the longitudinal arches of the foot.
    b. Check your text to confirm your information.
    c and d. Have your instructor confirm your accuracy.

25. Anterior talofibular, posterior talofibular, and calcaneofibular ligaments.

26. The anterior talofibular ligament.

*27. a. The deltoid ligament is designed to control distraction of the talus from the tibia and hold the calcaneus and navicular against the talus. The spring ligament assists in maintaining the medial longitudinal arch of the foot.
    b. Check your text to confirm your information.
    c, d, and e. Have your instructor confirm your accuracy.

28. a. Eversion.
    b. No.
    c. Because of the strength of the ligament, fracture of the malleolus rather than tearing of the ligament is more likely.

29. The attachments are the heads of the metatarsals, and the ligament helps maintain the transverse arch of the foot.

30. Medial longitudinal arch
    Bones involved: talus, calcaneus, navicular, three cuneiforms, and three metatarsal bones
    Major support: spring (plantar calcaneonavicular) ligament
    Lateral longitudinal arch
    Bones involved: calcaneus, cuboid, and the lateral two metatarsals
    Major support: long plantar ligament, short plantar ligament, and plantar aponeurosis
    Transverse arch
    Bones involved: cuboid, three cuneiforms, and metatarsals
    Major support: bony structure, the peroneus longus muscle, and deep transverse metatarsal ligament

31. Use your text to confirm your drawing. Since the plantar fascia begins at the calcaneus, crosses plantar to the MP joints, and is attached to the proximal phalanges, extension of the MP joints during gait increases the tension of the fascia and adds stability to the medial and lateral longitudinal arches.

*32. Use this exercise to gain an appreciation for the range of normal, and perhaps to see some abnormal arches of the feet. The navicular tubercle should fall on or close to the line that you drew. If it falls above the line and is pathological, it is called pes cavus; if it is below the line, it is pes planus. The ligamentous structures responsible for supporting the medial longitudinal arch are the long and short plantar ligaments, the spring ligament, and the plantar aponeurosis. In addition to ligamentous support, the bones themselves help support the arches. Muscles contribute relatively little to the support of the arches.

33. Tibialis posterior
    O: Medial surface of proximal two thirds of fibula; interosseous membrane; posterolateral surface of tibia
    I: Tuberosity of navicular; plantar surfaces of sustentaculum of calcaneus; cuneiforms; cuboid; bases of second, third, and fourth metatarsals
    N: Tibial n. (L-5, S-1)

R: Medial to axis for inversion and eversion; posterior to axis for plantarflexion

A: Plantarflexion, inversion

34. Peroneus longus

O: Proximal two thirds of lateral surface of fibula

I: Lateral aspect of base of first metatarsal and medial cuneiform

N: Superficial peroneal n. (L-4, L-5, S-1)

R: Lateral to axis for inversion and eversion; posterior to axis for dorsiflexion and plantarflexion

A: Eversion and plantarflexion

35. Peroneus brevis

O: Distal two thirds of lateral surface of fibula

I: Lateral aspect of base of fifth metatarsal

N: Superficial peroneal n. (L-4, L-5, S-1)

R: Lateral to axis for inversion and eversion; posterior to axis for dorsiflexion and plantarflexion

A: Eversion and plantarflexion

36. Tibialis anterior

O: Superior two thirds of lateral surface of tibia

I: Medial surface of first cuneiform; base of first metatarsal

N: Deep peroneal n. (L-4, L-5, S-1)

R: Anterior to axis for dorsiflexion and plantarflexion; medial to axis for inversion and eversion

A: Dorsiflexion and inversion

37. Extensor digitorum longus

O: Superior three quarters of anterior surface of fibula and lateral condyle of tibia

I: Divides into four tendons which insert onto the middle and distal phalanges of the lateral four digits

N: Deep peroneal n. (L-4, L-5, S-1)

R: Anterior to axis for flexion and extension; anterior to axis for ankle dorsiflexion and plantarflexion

A: Extension of lateral four toes and ankle dorsiflexion

38. Extensor digitorum brevis

O: Dorsal surface of calcaneus

I: Divides into four tendons which insert into the proximal phalanx of great toe and tendons of extensor digitorum longus of the second, third, and fourth toes

N: Deep peroneal n. (L-5, S-1)

R: Anterior to axis for flexion and extension

A: Extension of medial four toes

39. Extensor hallucis longus

O: Middle third of anterior surface of fibula

I: Base of distal phalanx of great toe

N: Deep peroneal n. (L-4, L-5, S-1)

R: Dorsal to axis for extension and flexion; anterior to axis for dorsiflexion and plantarflexion of foot

A: Extension of great toe and dorsiflexion of ankle

40. Gastrocnemius

O: Medial head: proximal and posterior aspect of medial condyle of femur
Lateral head: lateral condyle of femur

I: Tendocalcaneus which attaches to proximal posterior surface of calcaneus

N: Tibial n. (S-1, S-2)

R: Posterior to the axes for ankle plantarflexion and dorsiflexion and knee flexion and extension

A: Plantarflexion of ankle

*41. Soleus

    O: Posterior surface of head and shaft of fibula and body; middle third of medial tibia

    I: Tendocalcaneus (see gastrocnemius)

    N: Tibial n. (S-1, S-2)

    R: Posterior to the axis for plantarflexion and dorsiflexion of the ankle

    A: Plantarflexion of ankle

42. Plantaris

    O: Distal part of supracondylar line of femur

    I: Tendocalcaneus (see gastrocnemius)

    N: Tibial n. (S-1, S-2)

    R: Posterior to the axis for ankle plantarflexion and dorsiflexion

    A: Plantarflexion

43. Flexor digitorum brevis

    O: Calcaneus

    I: Middle phalanges of lateral four toes

    N: Medial plantar n. (L-4, L-5)

    R: Plantar to axis for flexion and extension

    A: Flexion of lateral four toes

44. Abductor hallucis

    O: Flexor retinaculum and calcaneus

    I: Base of proximal phalanx of great toe

    N: Medial plantar n. (S-2, S-3)

    R: Lateral and proximal to the axis for great toe abduction and adduction

    A: Abduction of great toe

45. Flexor hallucis longus

    O: Lower two thirds of posterior fibula

    I: Base of distal phalanx of great toe

    N: Tibial n. (L-5, S-1, S-2)

    R: Plantar to axis for flexion and extension

    A: Flexion of great toe

46. Flexor digitorum longus

    O: Posterior aspect of tibia

    I: Four tendons insert on the distal phalanges of lateral four digits

    N: Tibial n. (L-5, S-1)

    R: Posterior to axis for plantarflexion and dorsiflexion; plantar to axis for flexion and extension of the toes

    A: Flexion of lateral four toes and plantarflexion of ankle

47. See item 32, above.

48. See item 31, above.

49. With the knee flexed and the foot plantarflexed, the gastrocnemius generates less force (is weaker) due to active insufficiency. This, therefore, could provide a good position for ruling out the gastrocnemius when you want to assess the strength of the soleus.

50. The gastrocnemius can be stretched effectively by simultaneously causing knee extension and ankle dorsiflexion.

51. a. Helpful instructions for getting an isolated contraction of the tibialis anterior might be to give the subject a goal to touch, placed appropriately to achieve the muscle action wanted, i.e., dorsiflexion with inversion, as you say, "Touch my hand with your big toe."

b. Helpful instructions for getting an isolated contraction of the extensor hallucis longus might be "Let your foot hang loosely while you try gently to raise your big toe. Do not raise your other toes."

c. Helpful instructions for getting an isolated contraction of the extensor digitorum longus might be "Let your foot hang loosely while you try gently to raise your toes without raising your big toe."

NOTE: To get an isolated contraction, you may need to instruct your subject to try gently or easily so that he does not activate any muscles other than the one you are after.

52. With inversion sprains of the ankle, the peroneal muscles are stretched. This overstretching may cause weakening of the muscles. Strengthening these muscles may also help prevent reinjury to the area by strengthening the muscles that would resist inversion.

*53. a. This puts the foot in a toe-out position. Normal tibial torsion rotates the medial/lateral axis of the ankle joint to a line that is anterior medially and posterior laterally; by externally rotating the tibia further, this position is accentuated.

b. This puts the foot in a neutral or toe-in position. This puts the axis in a plane closer to the frontal plane or a reverse position to that of the previous activity.

c. The foot remains in the same position in relation to the supporting surface. In relation to the tibia, though, the foot is now more in a position of toe-in. The other joints of the foot will adjust to allow the sole of the foot to maintain contact with the floor. The medial longitudinal arch will be elevated, subtalar and transverse tarsal joints supinated, and the tarsometatarsal joints placed in a pronated twist to keep the toes in contact with the floor. The knee and hip will also be affected by this rotation of the tibia.

d. The foot remains in the same position in relation to the supporting surface. In relation to the tibia, though, the foot is now more in a position of toe-out. The other joints of the foot will adjust to allow the sole of the foot to maintain contact with the floor. This position will tend to depress the medial longitudinal arch, pronate the subtalar and transverse tarsal joints and place the tarsometatarsal joints in a supinated twist to keep the toes in contact with the ground. The knee and hip will also be affected by this rotation of the tibia.

*54. Seeing the closed-chain activity on a normal pliable foot is particularly instructive once you are aware of what you are looking for. The twist of the forefoot during closed-chain rotation of the tibia can be more readily observed on the normal foot than on an articulated model, since the models are not usually as pliable.

*55. This activity demonstrates the effect of varied foot position on the superimposed tibia. Again, the motions are closed-chain because the foot is on the ground.

a. Closed-chain pronation is accomplished by eversion of the calcaneus but adduction (medial rotation) and plantarflexion of the talus. Since the talus medially rotates, it will take the tibia with it and the tibia medially rotates.

b. The knee tends to assume a greater valgus posture as a result of closed-chain pronation of the foot.

*56. With severe pes planus, the navicular and the head of the talus come in contact with the ground. The calcaneus and transtarsal joints are pronated. This causes genu valgus. Over a prolonged period of time, this pathology may lead to hip degeneration and low back problems because of the prolonged application of abnormal forces through the knees.

*57. Check with a text and confirm your information with a faculty member.

*58. The fifth metatarsal and the sole of the foot are not parallel. Therefore, if the sole of the foot is parallel to the floor, the fifth metatarsal cannot be. The implication for goniometry is that the two different referents cannot be used interchangeably. Either referent (head and base of fifth metatarsal or sole of foot) can be used, but different readings will be obtained.

*59. Use this activity to explore the range of normal.

*60. In most individuals, you will find increased dorsiflexion with knee flexion. By flexing the knee, the gastrocnemius is put on slack and will not limit dorsiflexion. When the knee is extended and the ankle dorsiflexed, the gastrocnemius may be passively insufficient.

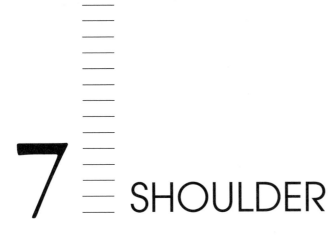

7 ≡ SHOULDER

OSTEOLOGY OF THE SHOULDER

The shoulder complex allows great mobility in the upper extremity, but at the expense of stability. Its articulations are loose, allowing the bones a wide range of motion.

1. What are the bones of the shoulder complex? (Ignore the ribs for now.)

*2. Identify the following landmarks on a skeleton, then palpate as many of them as possible on a partner. Locate all of them on Figures 7-1 to 7-3.

Scapula
Inferior angle
Superior angle
Medial border
Lateral border
Coracoid process
Spine
Glenoid fossa
Infraglenoid tubercle
Supraglenoid tubercle
Acromion

Clavicle
Sternal end
Anterior concavity
Acromial end

Humerus
Head
Anatomical neck
Surgical neck
Greater tubercle
Lesser tubercle
Bicipital groove
Deltoid tuberosity

Sternum
Sternal notch
Xyphoid process

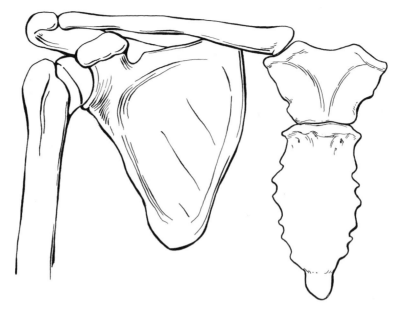

FIGURE 7–1

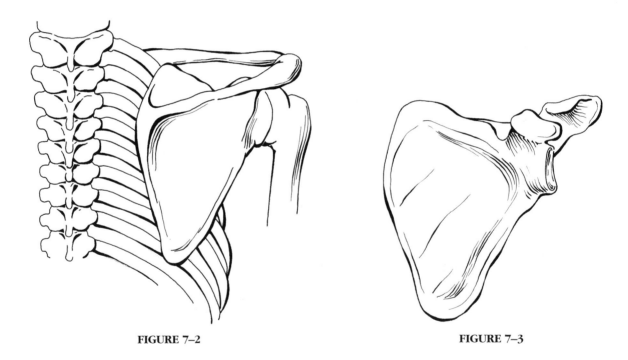

FIGURE 7–2

FIGURE 7–3

3. Describe the orientation of the surface of the glenoid fossa in relationship to the trunk when the shoulder girdle is in the normal resting position. You may need an accurately articulated skeleton to aid in this description.

4. Discuss the relative congruence of the humeral head and glenoid fossa. Hint: Look at the size and shape of
each. In your discussion, include the relationship of congruence to stability of the glenohumeral joint.

ARTHROLOGY OF THE SHOULDER

The articulations of the shoulder complex are:

Diarthrodial joints:
   Sternoclavicular
   Acromioclavicular
   Glenohumeral

Functional joints:
   Scapulothoracic
   Coracoacromial arch

Fill in the necessary information about the joints and articulations in the outline and diagrams below.

Sternoclavicular Joint

5. Give the type of diarthrodial joint, number of degrees of freedom of movement, and movements available at the sternoclavicular joint. How are the names of the movements determined?

6. Label each of the following ligaments on Figure 7–4:

   Interclavicular ligament
   Costoclavicular ligament
   Anterior sternoclavicular ligaments

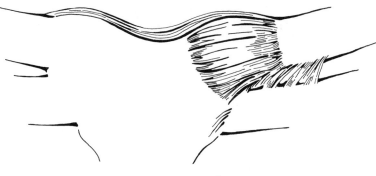

FIGURE 7–4

7. Give a description and discuss the role of the articular disc of the sternoclavicular (SC) joint.

8. Give the function (control of motion or stabilization) of each of the ligaments associated with the sternoclavicular joint.

a. Interclavicular

b. Costoclavicular

c. Anterior and posterior sternoclavicular

*9. Perform the following clavicular motions yourself, then observe them on a partner. Beside each motion, note what extremity or scapular motion was required to produce the clavicular motion.

a. Elevation: _____

_____

b. Depression: _____

_____

c. Protraction: _____

_____

d. Retraction: _____

_____

e. Rotation: _____

_____

Acromioclavicular Joint

10. Give the type of joint and number of degrees of freedom of movement at the acromioclavicular joint. In your own words, give the motions of the scapula at the acromioclavicular joint.

11. Label each of the following ligaments on Figure 7-5:

Coracoclavicular ligament
Acromioclavicular ligament
Coracoacromial ligament

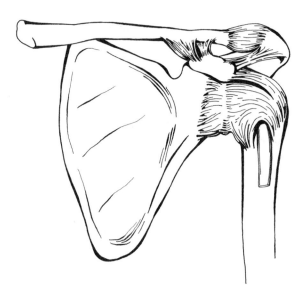

FIGURE 7–5

12. Give the function (control of motion or stabilization) of each of the ligaments associated with the acromioclavicular joint.

   a. Coracoclavicular
      Conoid portion

      Trapezoid portion

   b. Acromioclavicular

   c. Coracoacromial

Glenohumeral Joint

13. Give the type of joint and number of degrees of freedom of the glenohumeral joint.

14. On Figure 7-5 in item 11, label the following ligaments of the glenohumeral joint:
    Glenohumeral ligament
    Coracohumeral ligament

*15. Select a subject with her back exposed. Stabilize the right scapula with your right hand on the lateral border so that it does not move laterally during abduction or flexion of the humerus at the shoulder. Ask the subject to flex the humerus at the shoulder. Make sure the scapula does not move. Then ask her to abduct the humerus at the shoulder. Again, make sure that the scapula does not move. Now, repeat the motions and allow the scapula to participate in each of the movements freely.

   Now, press your hand on the flat of the scapula so that the inferior angle of the scapula maintains close contact with the chest wall. Ask the subject to rotate the humerus medially at the shoulder with the scapula stabilized and then with it free to move.

   Describe the difference in range of motion available in all of these situations.

*16. Describe the movement of the humeral head on the glenoid fossa during abduction of the humerus at the shoulder.

17. During abduction of the humerus, what force keeps the humeral head from rolling superiorly off the glenoid fossa?

*18. This activity is best done with the subject supine. Be sure that your partner does not have an unstable shoulder; then place her left shoulder in the abducted, externally rotated position with the shoulder at the edge of the treatment table. Hold her left elbow in your left hand with her elbow bent at an acute angle. Place the fingertips of your right hand posterior to the head of the humerus so that you can push it anteriorly, and support her left forearm with your right forearm. You are testing for anterior glenohumeral instability. To perform the test, abduct the humerus 60° away from the side of the chest wall; then simultaneously press the proximal humerus anteriorly with the fingers of your right hand while you horizontally adduct the humerus with your left hand allowing her forearm to rest on your right forearm. Bring the humerus back to the 60° abducted position and move to 90°. Repeat the procedure of horizontal adduction while pressing the proximal humerus forward. Repeat the procedure again starting at 120° of abduction. If the joint were unstable, you would feel the head of the humerus relocating into the glenoid as you horizontally adduct. This means that the anterior pressure from your right hand was sufficient to displace the head at least slightly out of the glenoid. We hope that your classmate's shoulder does not demonstrate this level of instability. What passive structure prevents the excessive anterior shift in each of the positions (60°, 90°, and 120°) in your subject?

19. Describe the major bursa of the shoulder joint associated with abduction of the humerus at the shoulder and give its main functions.

20. Give the attachments for the joint capsule of the glenohumeral joint. Describe the capsule's outstanding features and the functional implications of those features.

Scapulothoracic Joint

21. Name the motions of the scapula, giving all the synonyms for the motions that occur in various readings such as your kinesiology text, muscle-testing text, anatomy text, and goniometry text.

22. Describe, in your own words, scapulohumeral rhythm.

23. Which of the joints of the shoulder girdle is the only bony attachment of the shoulder girdle to the trunk?

MYOLOGY OF THE SHOULDER

Use the following muscle sheets to aid in learning the origins, insertions, and innervations of the shoulder muscles. For each of the muscles named, draw in the muscle on the sketch and complete the indicated information in the outline.

O: Origin of muscle
I: Insertion of muscle
N: Innervation (both peripheral nerve and spinal level)
R: Relationship of muscle to axis of motion
A: Action of muscle

24. Pectoralis major

O: Anterior surface of clavicle, sternum
I: Greater tubercle of humerus
N: Medial and lateral pectoral n. (C-5, C-6, C-7, C-8, T-1)
R: Fibers run obliquely and horizontally; medial (or inferior) to axis for abduction and adduction; anterior and wraps around longitudinally to axis for medial rotation; medial to axis for horizontal abduction and adduction
A: Adduction, horizontal adduction, and medial rotation of the humerus at the shoulder

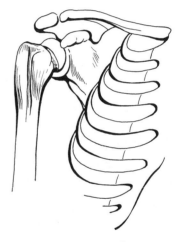

FIGURE 7–6

25. Pectoralis minor

O:
I:
N: Medial pectoral n. (C-6, C-7, C-8, T-1)
R: Fibers run upward and obliquely from medial to lateral
A: Downward scapular rotation and anterior tipping of the scapula

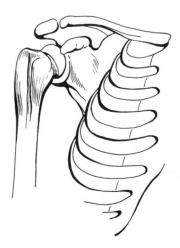

FIGURE 7–6

26. Serratus anterior

    O: Outer superior border of first 8–9 ribs
    I:
    N:
    R: Line of force runs from anterior on the thorax to posterior on the medial border of the scapula
    A: Scapular abduction (protraction); some upward rotation of scapula

27. Coracobrachialis

    O: Coracoid process
    I: Middle third of the medial surface of the shaft of the humerus
    N: Musculocutaneous n. (C-6, C-7)
    R:
    A: Shoulder flexion and slight adduction

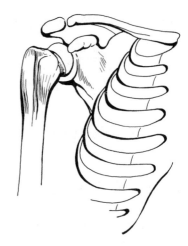

FIGURE 7–6

28. Subscapularis

    O: Subscapular fossa
    I:
    N: Upper and lower subscapular n. (C-5, C-6)
    R:
    A: Medial rotation of the humerus at the shoulder and assists in stabilizing the head of the humerus on the glenoid fossa during humeral elevation

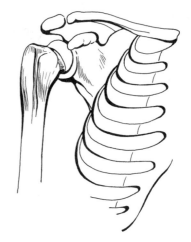

FIGURE 7–6

29. Supraspinatus

    O: Supraspinous fossa of the scapula
    I:
    N: Suprascapular n. (C-4, C-5, C-6)
    R:
    A: Abduction of the humerus at the shoulder; assists in stabilizing the head of the humerus on the glenoid fossa during humeral elevation

30. Teres minor

    O:
    I: Lowest point of greater tubercle of humerus
    N:
    R: Obliquely upward from O to I; wraps around longitudinal axis posterolaterally
    A: Lateral rotation and extension of the humerus at the shoulder, assists in stabilizing the head of the humerus on the glenoid fossa during humeral elevation

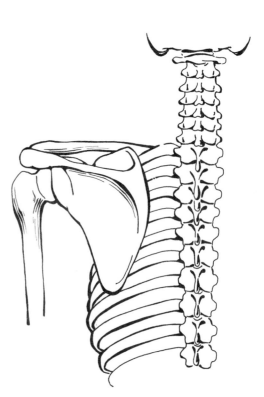

FIGURE 7–7

31. Infraspinatus

   O:

   I: Middle point of greater tubercle of humerus

   N: Suprascapular n. (C-4, C-5, C-6)

   R:

   A: Lateral rotation of the humerus at the shoulder, assists in stabilizing the head of the humerus on the glen-oid fossa during humeral elevation

32. Teres major

   O:

   I: Inferior to lesser tuberosity of humerus, posterior to latissimus dorsi

   N: Lower subscapular n. (C-5, C-6, C-7)

   R:

   A: Extension, adduction, medial rotation of the humerus at the shoulder

33. Levator scapulae

   O: Transverse processes of atlas, axis, and 3 to 4 of the cervical vertebrae

   I:

   N: Branch of dorsal scapular n. (C-3, C-4)

   R: Slightly oblique from superior and medial O to inferior and lateral I

   A: Scapular elevation

34. Rhomboids

   O:

   I:

   N: Dorsal scapular n. (C-4, C-5)

   R:

   A: Scapular retraction (adduction) with downward rotation

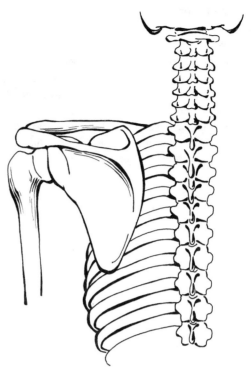

FIGURE 7–7

35. Latissimus dorsi

    O:

    I:

    N: Thoracodorsal n. (C-6, C-7, C-8)

    R: Fibers run inferior to superior from medial O to lateral I; posterior to axis for flexion and extension; wraps medially around the axis for rotation; medial (or inferior) to axis for abduction and adduction

    A: Extension, medial rotation, adduction of the humerus at the shoulder

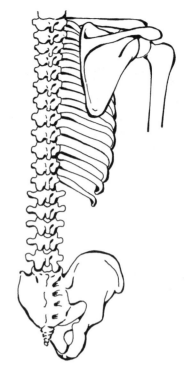

FIGURE 7–8

36. Deltoid

    O:

    I: Deltoid tuberosity of humerus

    N:

    R: Anterior fibers—slightly oblique, superior to inferior, and anterior to the axis for flexion and extension;

    Posterior fibers—slightly oblique, superior to inferior, and posterior to the axis for flexion and extension;

    Middle fibers—straight from superior to inferior, and lateral (or superior) to the axis for abduction and adduction

    A: Anterior fibers—flexion of the humerus at the shoulder; horizontal adduction of the humerus at the shoulder;

    Posterior fibers—extension of the humerus at the shoulder; horizontal abduction of the humerus at the shoulder;

    Middle fibers—abduction of the humerus at the shoulder

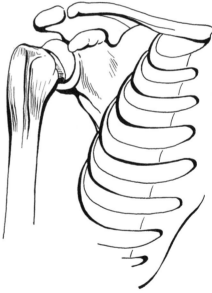

FIGURE 7–6

37. Trapezius
    O: Upper fibers—from the external occipital protuber-
       ance; medial third of the nuchal line; the ligamen-
       tum nuchae; and the posterior spinous process of
       the seventh cervical vertebra;
       Middle fibers—from the posterior spinous
       processes of the first through fifth thoracic verte-
       brae;
       Lower fibers—from the posterior spinous
       processes of the 6th through 12th thoracic verte-
       brae
     I: Upper fibers—to the lateral third of the clavicle
       and the acromion;
       Middle fibers—to the acromion and spine of the
       scapula;
       Lower fibers—to the vertebral end of the spine of
       the scapula
    N:
    R:
    A:

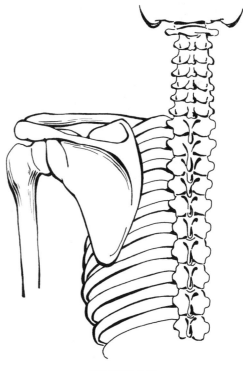

FIGURE 7–7

38. For the arm to move accurately in space, it must work from a stable base, in this case a stable scapula. List the muscles that stabilize the scapula on the thorax.

39. Make a list of the muscles whose lines of pull could each produce an inferior glide of the head of the humerus on the surface of the glenoid fossa. Which of these muscles actively participate with the humeral elevators during elevation of the hand above the head?

40. Which of the scapular stabilizers can perform upward rotation of the scapula?

41. What muscles can produce motion at both the shoulder and the elbow with the arm in an open kinematic chain?

42. Give the most likely antagonist for each of the following muscles:
    a. Posterior deltoid _____
    b. Serratus anterior _____
    c. Rhomboids _____
    d. Teres major _____
    e. Pectoralis minor _____

APPLICATIONS

*43. Using an articulated skeleton, examine the relationship of the greater tuberosity and the acromion during abduction without rotation of the humerus at the shoulder. What occurs with this relationship if the humerus is medially rotated during abduction? Laterally rotated?

*44. Place your subject supine on the plinth with her shoulder at the edge of the plinth. Stand on the side of the plinth near that shoulder and support the upper extremity by holding the subject's hand. Try to get your subject completely relaxed so that you can move the extremity passively with no participation from the subject's musculature. Be sure to have the extremity high enough to clear the humerus from the plinth surface. Now, *passively* move the extremity into complete abduction. Be sure to move slowly and continue to obtain complete relaxation from the subject. At the beginning of the movement, you should see the anterior surface of the brachium uppermost. At the end of the range of motion, you should see the medial surface of the brachium uppermost. (Uppermost means facing toward the ceiling.)

   Describe the motion of the humerus at the glenohumeral joint that you observed. Considering that there was no muscle contraction on the part of the subject and that you did not try to create any motion other than abduction, explain why this motion occurred. Hint: Examine the configuration of the fibers of the articular capsule.

*45. Have your subject perform active extension of the humerus at the shoulder in a fashion that will allow the triceps to assist with the movement with the greatest active tension possible through the largest range of motion possible. What principle was being demonstrated?

*46. Your partner has lost function of cranial nerve XI. Muscle-test the muscles directly affected, and then the glenohumeral movements secondarily affected.

*47. Reverse action is typically the moving of the origin toward the insertion. That means that the insertion becomes the stable point. This is so even when the origin is on the trunk and the insertion is on the humerus or scapula. To demonstrate, either you or your partner perform the reverse actions of the following muscles:

   a. Latissimus dorsi
   b. Lower trapezius
   c. Pectoralis major, lower fibers

      Of what clinical significance is the ability to perform these reverse actions?

*48. Examine the scapulohumeral rhythm of your partner and decide at what point in the active range of abduction of the humerus at the shoulder the scapula first begins upward rotation. Record the goniometric value of humeral elevation at that point. Have your partner repeat this process with you. Compare the two values. How similar or different were the values? How do they compare to standard values you have found in texts for the point at which the scapula begins to move?

*49. Actively fix (hold still with your muscles) the glenohumeral joint so that no motion occurs there. Maintain the fixation and move your upper extremity away from your body. What movements did you use to accomplish the activity? How do your observations apply to accurate manual muscle testing and goniometry of the shoulder?

*50. Position the upper extremity to place the long head of the triceps on maximum stretch.

*51. Repeat the procedure to stretch the long head of the biceps.

*52. Position the upper extremity in order to palpate the greater tuberosity of the humerus. What tendon becomes more superficial and accessible to treatment in this position?

53. What joint is primarily affected by the costoclavicular ligament? What are the effects on that joint of a torn costoclavicular ligament?

54. Tightness in the anterior portion of the capsule of the glenohumeral joint limits lateral rotation of the humerus at the shoulder. What additional motion of the glenohumeral joint can be limited as a result of the limited lateral rotation? Why?

55. Fracture of the greater tuberosity of the humerus directly affects the actions of what muscles? With these muscles effectively weakened, what shoulder motions are affected and what functional activities limited?

56. Examine the anatomy of the glenohumeral joint and decide what structures would be most disrupted by an anterior-inferior dislocation of the glenohumeral joint. What are two muscles that reinforce the anterior portion of the joint? Which would you think is the stronger reinforcer of the joint?

57. Describe the two force couples of the shoulder girdle that assist in elevation of the upper extremity above the head. Give the muscles involved in each and the function accomplished by each force couple.

ANSWERS TO SHOULDER

1. Seven bones make up the shoulder complex:

   Two scapulae
   Two clavicles
   Two humeri
   One sternum

2. The first eight scapular items, the last four humeral items, and all clavicular and sternal items should be palpable. Check your text and have a faculty member confirm your information.

3. The glenoid fossa faces anteriorly, laterally, and superiorly in the resting shoulder girdle.

4. The humeral head is disproportionately large in relation to the glenoid fossa; the fossa is shallow. Both conditions create an unstable joint needing considerable stabilization from ligaments and muscles.

5. The sternoclavicular joint is a plane synovial joint with three degrees of freedom of movement. The movements are determined by the movement of the distal end of the clavicle and are:

   Elevation and depression
   Protraction and retraction
   Rotation

6. Check your text and have a faculty member confirm your information.

7. The SC joint disc is attached superiorly to the clavicle and inferiorly to the sternum and provides some congruity to the highly incongruous SC joint. It is interposed between the medial end of the clavicle and the sternum and allows for some contact between the superior half of the medial end of the clavicle and the sternum.

8. a. The interclavicular ligament limits depression of the clavicle.
   b. The costoclavicular ligament limits protraction, retraction, and also elevation of the clavicle.
   c. The anterior and posterior sternoclavicular ligaments reinforce the joint capsule and limit the anterior/posterior movement of the medial end of the clavicle that is associated with retraction and protraction. This movement of the medial end of the clavicle is due to the fact that the axis of rotation for protraction and retraction is through the costoclavicular ligament.

*9. a. Elevation of the clavicle accompanies scapular elevation.
   b. Depression of the clavicle accompanies scapular depression.
   c. Protraction of the clavicle accompanies scapular abduction.
   d. Retraction of the clavicle accompanies scapular adduction.
   e. Rotation of the clavicle occurs after the clavicle has completed its elevation and accompanies upward rotation of the scapula.

10. The acromioclavicular joint is a plane synovial joint with three degrees of freedom. The scapular movements include rotation in the frontal plane, winging in the horizontal plane, and tipping in the sagittal plane.

11. Check your text and, if necessary, have a faculty member confirm your information.

12. a. The coracoclavicular ligament helps maintain the integrity of the acromioclavicular joint by holding the clavicle to the coracoid process. The trapezoid portion pulls the clavicle into backward rotation as a result of scapular upward rotation that occurs past 90° of humeral elevation.
   b. The acromioclavicular ligament maintains apposition of the joint surfaces and helps prevent posterior dislocation of the clavicle on the acromion.
   c. The coracoacromial ligament closes the coracoacromial arch and prevents superior dislocation of the humeral head.

13. The glenohumeral joint is a ball-and-socket joint with three degrees of freedom of movement.

14. Check your text and have a faculty member confirm your information.

15. In all cases where you have manually prevented scapular movement, the humeral excursion will be less than normally expected. Full motion of the humerus requires simultaneous scapular motion.

16. Abduction of the humerus at the shoulder produces superior rolling and inferior gliding of the head of the humerus.

17. The inferiorly directed force of the rotator cuff muscles counteracts the superior rolling of the humeral head.

*18. a. The superior, middle, and inferior bands of the glenohumeral ligament provide the anterior stabilization in the 60°, 90°, and 120° positions respectively, assuming that the subject is relaxed. You will need a good atlas of anatomy with the shoulder ligaments well identified to be able to visualize this information.

19. The subacromial/subdeltoid bursa is a synovial sac with potential space that extends from below the acromion to the lateral aspect of the humerus. It is superficial to the tendon of the supraspinatus and deep to the deltoid muscle. It assists in providing smooth sliding of the greater tuberosity under the acromion during humeral elevation.

20. The capsule of the glenohumeral joint attaches medially around the glenoid fossa proximal to the labrum, extends to the root of the coracoid process enclosing the proximal attachment of the biceps long head, and attaches laterally at the anatomical neck of the humerus, extending a sleeve along the bicipital groove surrounding the biceps long-head tendon in the groove. The capsule is large and loose, providing great range of motion, and the inferior portion lies in folds when the humerus is at rest in upright posture. The inferior portion is the weakest portion of the fibrous capsule.

21. The motions of the scapula include elevation, depression, abduction (protraction), adduction (retraction), upward rotation, downward rotation, anterior tipping (rounding), posterior tipping (opposite of rounding), and winging (medial border of the scapula comes away from the chest wall).

22. Since the description is in your own words, it is impossible to give the *correct* answer here. However, you should include the aspects of humeral elevation with scapular upward rotation and humeral lowering with scapular downward rotation as well as the ratio of humeral movement to scapular movement. Also discuss the effect the scapular movement has on the length-tension relationship of the deltoid and its effect on joint congruity in the glenohumeral joint.

23. The sternoclavicular joint is the only bony attachment of the shoulder girdle to the trunk.

24. Pectoralis major, all items given in text.

25. Pectoralis minor.
    O: Anterior and superior margins of the third, fourth, and fifth ribs
    I: Coracoid process of the scapula
    N: Medial pectoral n. (C-6, C-7, C-8, T-1)
    R: Fibers run upward and obliquely from medial to lateral
    A: Downward scapular rotation and anterior tipping of the scapula

26. Serratus anterior
    O: Outer superior border of first 8 to 9 ribs
    I: Ventral surface of medial border of scapula
    N: Long thoracic n. (C-5, C-6, C-7, C-8)
    R: Line of force runs from anterior on the thorax to posterior on the medial border of the scapula
    A: Scapular abduction and some upward rotation of scapula

27. Coracobrachialis
    O: Coracoid process of the scapula
    I: Middle third of the medial surface of the shaft of the humerus

N: Musculocutaneous n. (C-6, C-7)

R: Slightly oblique from O to I and anterior to axis for shoulder flexion and extension

A: Flexion of the humerus at the shoulder and slight adduction

28. Subscapularis

O: Subscapular fossa

I: Lesser tubercle of the humerus and the joint capsule

N: Upper and lower subscapular n. (C-5, C-6)

R: Slightly oblique from O to I and anterior to the axis for rotation of the humerus at the shoulder

A: Medial rotation of the humerus at the shoulder and assists in stabilizing the head of the humerus on the glenoid fossa during humeral elevation

29. Supraspinatus

O: Supraspinous fossa of the scapula

I: Highest point of greater tubercle of humerus

N: Suprascapular n. (C-4, C-5, C-6)

R: Straight (horizontal) from O to I and superior and lateral to axis for abduction and adduction

A: Abduction of the humerus at the shoulder and assists in stabilizing the head of the humerus on the glenoid fossa during humeral elevation

30. Teres minor

O: Axillary border of scapula

I: Lowest point of greater tubercle of humerus

N: Axillary n. (C-5, C-6)

R: Obliquely upward from O to I; wraps around longitudinal axis posteriolaterally

A: Lateral rotation and extension of the humerus at the shoulder and assists in stabilizing the head of the humerus on the glenoid fossa during humeral elevation

31. Infraspinatus

O: Infraspinous fossa

I: Middle point of greater tubercle of humerus

N: Suprascapular n. (C-4, C-5, C-6)

R: Upward, oblique from O to I and wraps around laterally to the longitudinal axis

A: Lateral rotation of the humerus at the shoulder and assists in stabilizing the head of the humerus on the glenoid fossa during humeral elevation

32. Teres major

O: Inferior angle of scapula

I: Inferior to lesser tuberosity of humerus; posterior to latissimus dorsi

N: Lower subscapular n. (C-5, C-6, C-7)

R: Oblique, superiorly from O to I and wraps medially to the longitudinal axis; medial (or inferior) to the axis for adduction and abduction; posterior to the axis for flexion and extension

A: Extension, adduction, medial rotation of the humerus at the shoulder

33. Levator scapulae

O: Transverse processes of atlas, axis, and 3 to 4 of the cervical vertebrae

I: Vertebral border of scapula, superior to root of spine

N: Branch of dorsal scapular n. (C-3, C-4)

R: Slightly oblique from superior and medial O to inferior and lateral I

A: Scapular elevation and downward rotation

34. Rhomboids

O: Spinous processes C-7 to T-5

I: Vertebral border of scapula from spine to inferior angle

N: Dorsal scapular n. (C-4, C-5)

R: Oblique from superior to inferior from O to I and posterior and medial to the axis for adduction and abduction of the scapula

A: Scapular retraction (adduction) with downward rotation

35. Latissimus dorsi

O: Spines of lower six thoracic, lumbar, and sacral vertebrae; posterior aspect of iliac crest; three or four lower ribs; and perhaps the inferior angle of the scapula

I: Intertubercular groove of humerus

N: Thoracodorsal n. (C-6, C-7, C-8)

R: Fibers run inferior to superior from medial O to lateral I; posterior to axis for flexion and extension; wrap medially around the axis for rotation; medial (or inferior) to the axis for abduction and adduction

A: Extension, medial rotation, adduction of the humerus at the shoulder

36. Deltoid

O: Anterior border, superior surface of the lateral third of clavicle (anterior fibers); lateral margin and superior surface of the acromion (middle fibers); inferior lip of the posterior border of the spine of the scapula (posterior fibers)

I: Deltoid tubercle of humerus

N: Axillary n. (C-5, C-6)

R: Anterior fibers—slightly oblique, superior to inferior and anterior to the axis for flexion and extension; Posterior fibers—slightly oblique, superior to inferior and posterior to the axis for flexion and extension; Middle fibers—straight from superior to inferior and lateral to the axis for abduction and adduction

A: Anterior fibers—flexion of the humerus at the shoulder; horizontal adduction of the humerus at the shoulder; Posterior fibers—extension of the humerus at the shoulder; horizontal abduction of the humerus at the shoulder; Middle fibers—abduction of the humerus at the shoulder

37. Trapezius

O: Upper fibers—external occipital protuberance; medial third of the nuchal line; the ligamentum nuchae; and the posterior spinous process of the seventh cervical vertebra; Middle fibers—posterior spinous processes of the first through fifth thoracic vertebrae; Lower fibers—posterior spinous processes of the sixth through twelfth thoracic vertebrae

I: Upper fibers—lateral third of the clavicle and the acromion; Middle fibers—acromion and spine of the scapula; Lower fibers—vertebral end of the spine of the scapula

N: Spinal accessory n. (cranial n. XI)

R: Upper fibers run obliquely and laterally from superior to inferior, superior to the axis for elevation; Middle fibers run horizontally from O to I, medial to the axis for adduction and abduction; Lower fibers run obliquely and laterally from inferior O to superior I, inferior to the axis for depression

A: Upper fibers—scapular elevation; upward rotation; Middle fibers—scapular retraction (adduction); Lower fibers—scapular depression, adduction, and upward rotation

38. The primary muscles that stabilize the scapula on the thorax are those that have attachments to each—that is, trapezius (all portions), levator scapulae, rhomboids, serratus anterior, pectoralis minor.

39. The muscles that could produce an inferior glide of the humeral head on the glenoid fossa would have a line of pull that runs from inferior to superior and from either the scapula or thorax to the humerus—that is, latissimus dorsi, teres major, teres minor, infraspinatus, subscapularis, and pectoralis major (sternal fibers). The ones that participate with the humeral elevators are the teres minor, infraspinatus, and subscapularis.

40. The scapular stabilizers that also produce some upward rotation of the scapula are the upper trapezius, lower trapezius, and serratus anterior.

41. The only two-joint muscles at the shoulder and elbow are the biceps and the triceps (long head).

42. a. Antagonists to the posterior deltoid: Anterior deltoid opposes extension of the humerus at the shoulder; pectoralis major opposes horizontal abduction
   b. Antagonist to the serratus anterior: Rhomboids oppose scapular abduction and upward rotation
   c. Antagonist to the rhomboids: Serratus anterior opposes scapular adduction and downward rotation
   d. Antagonist to the teres major: Teres minor opposes medial rotation of the humerus at the shoulder; middle deltoid opposes adduction of the humerus at the shoulder; anterior deltoid opposes extension of the humerus at the shoulder
   e. Antagonist to the pectoralis minor: Lower trapezius opposes anterior tipping of the scapula

*43. This activity is designed to provide a visual reference for one aspect of the biomechanics of abduction of the humerus at the shoulder. The greater tuberosity abuts the acromion during pure abduction of the humerus at the shoulder. This contact occurs earlier in the range of motion if the humerus is medially rotated, and is avoided if it is laterally rotated during the abduction movement.

*44. This activity is designed to demonstrate the role of the glenohumeral joint capsule in providing the needed lateral rotation during abduction of the humerus at the shoulder. The learners will be able to understand the result more clearly if they consult an anatomy text showing the alignment of the capsule fibers. This activity also provides kinesthetic practice to the learners who are attempting to feel the difference between partial and complete relaxation on the part of the subject.

*45. This activity reinforces the principle of two-joint muscles maintaining strength of contraction through a wide range of movement. This is accomplished by preventing active insufficiency through compensatory lengthening at one joint while shortening at another joint. The participants should see the functional movement of combined shoulder extension with elbow flexion. These combined motions provide lengthening of the triceps long head over the elbow with shortening at the shoulder. This is the combined movement used in lifting a weight from the floor. The reciprocal relationship between the motions over two joints of a two-joint muscle is also demonstrated in the hamstrings and in the rectus femoris as discussed in the hip chapter (Chapter 4). Note that the biceps brachii also maintains a favorable length-tension relationship through combined shoulder extension and elbow flexion.

*46. The primary muscles to be tested are the trapezius and the sternocleidomastoid. Secondary muscles are related to the trapezius since it is a scapular stabilizer for humeral elevation. In this case, any muscle primarily responsible for humeral elevation would be tested.

*47. This activity reinforces the principle of reverse actions. In this case, the distal part is the humerus and scapula and the proximal part is the trunk. The learner stabilizes the humerus and scapula and elevates the trunk. A sitting push-up will accomplish all the reverse actions at once. One clinical significance of understanding this reverse action is understanding that these are some of the prime muscles used in crutch walking. There are many other clinically significant understandings available including the neurological levels needed to perform a sitting push-up, and so on.

*48. This activity allows for practice of shoulder goniometry, for palpation of joint and scapular motion, and for the appreciation of the variation in normal. Large discrepancies may be seen during this activity, and goniometric reliability and validity can also be discussed, as well as the value of accurate palpation and observation.

*49. This activity demonstrates the usual joint motion substitution pattern for tightness in the glenohumeral joint or weakness in a glenohumeral joint elevator muscle. The result will reinforce the value of stabilization when muscle-testing the elevators of the humerus at the shoulder as well as when doing goniometry of the glenohumeral joint. In both of these activities (muscle testing and goniometry), joint motion rather than movement of the shoulder complex is the intent of the evaluation.

*50. This activity reinforces the principle of flexibility testing or stretching of a two-joint muscle, and demonstrates the position of all joints necessary to demonstrate passive insufficiency in a two-joint muscle.

*51. See item 50.

*52. To expose the greater tuberosity for easy palpation, the humerus must be extended and medially rotated at the shoulder. The rotator cuff tendon is most accessible in this position.

53. A torn costoclavicular ligament will change the axis for protraction and retraction and for elevation and depression at the sternoclavicular joint. It will also allow translatory force to be transmitted directly from the scapula to the SC joint. The first consequence will be movement at the SC joint (medial end) in the same direction as movement at the distal (acromial) end, rather than the clavicle moving in one direction on the sternum and in a different direction at the distal end. The second consequence will be greater wear and tear on the joint than there would be if the ligament were intact.

54. Abduction of the humerus will also be limited, since lateral rotation is necessary for the greater tuberosity to clear the acromion.

55. Most rotator cuff muscles will be affected, thus affecting lateral rotation and abduction or elevation of the humerus. The rotation is obvious; the effect on abduction or elevation is because the rotator cuff must be effective in order to produce a force couple with the deltoid to produce strong rotary motion of the lever, in this case elevation of the humerus. If the counterforce of the rotator cuff is not effective, the deltoid will provide more translatory than rotary force.

56. The most likely structures damaged in an anterior-inferior dislocation of the shoulder would be the anterior capsule, the subscapularis muscle, and the biceps long-head tendon. Other structures frequently damaged are the anterior glenoid labrum and frequently the bony rim of the fossa. The two muscles have just been mentioned. The subscapularis has much greater mass than the biceps tendon, so we would expect it to have a larger role in stabilizing the joint.

57. The two force couples of the shoulder complex are the scapular upward rotation couple and the humeral elevation couple. The scapular force couple is composed of the upper and lower trapezius and the serratus anterior with the center of rotation being within the scapula, but at different points during the full excursion of range of motion. When all are working in concert, upward rotation occurs. The humeral force couple consists of the deltoid pulling up and the rotator cuff pulling down with the center of rotation between the greater tuberosity and the deltoid tubercle. Such a center of rotation will produce significant downward stabilization of the head on the glenoid fossa, thus preventing the greater tuberosity from impinging on the acromion. Rotation about this center will also produce elevation of the humerus.

8 ELBOW AND FOREARM

OSTEOLOGY OF THE ELBOW AND FOREARM

*1. Identify the following structures on a laboratory partner:

Medial and lateral epicondyle of humerus	Palmaris longus
Medial and lateral supracondylar line	Flexor carpi ulnaris
Olecranon process	Triceps (three heads)
Olecranon fossa	Biceps brachii
Ulnar border	Brachialis
Radial head	Brachioradialis
Ulnar nerve at elbow	Extensor carpi radialis longus and brevis
Muscle bellies:	Extensor carpi ulnaris
Pronator teres	Tendons of the biceps, brachialis, and triceps
Flexor carpi radialis	Brachial artery

*2. Label the bony landmarks or prominences indicated on Figures 8-1 to 8-3. Put a star by those that you can palpate. Make sure that you can find the starred ones on your laboratory partner.

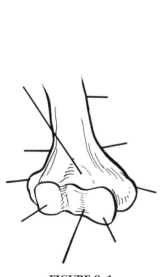

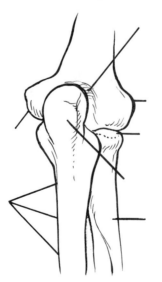

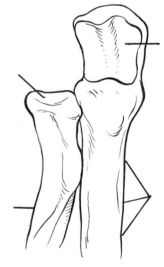

FIGURE 8–1   **FIGURE 8–2**   **FIGURE 8–3**

ARTHROLOGY OF THE ELBOW AND FOREARM

3. On Figures 8-4 to 8-6, draw in the annular ligament, radial collateral ligament, ulnar collateral ligament, and interosseous membrane.

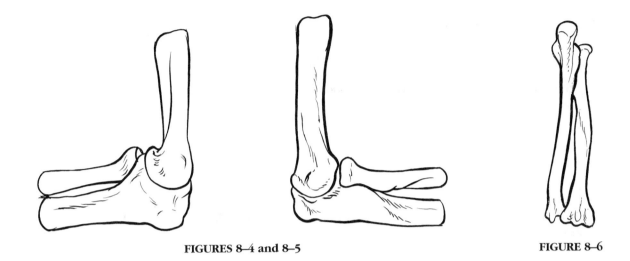

FIGURES 8–4 and 8–5   **FIGURE 8–6**

4. What is the function of the interosseous membrane? Why are the fibers of the interosseous membrane aligned as they are?

5. What is the function of the annular ligament?

6. Complete the following outline:

   Humeroulnar joint

      Type of joint

      Type of motion that occurs at joint

      Amount of motion available at joint (give the range of motion normally available and degrees of freedom)

7. Complete the following outline:
   Humeroradial joint
   > Type of joint

   > Type of motion that occurs at joint

8. Using the convex-concave rule, describe the motions of flexion and extension of the forearm at the humero-ulnar and humeroradial joints.

*9. On a laboratory partner, compare the end-feels of flexion and extension of the elbow. The two should feel different. What normally limits these two motions? How would you explain the difference in the end-feels?

10. Complete the following outline:
    Proximal radioulnar joint
    > Type of joint

    > Type of motion that occurs at joint

11. Complete the following outline:
    Distal radioulnar joint
    > Type of joint

    > Type of motion that occurs at joint

12. The radioulnar joints are involved in what motions? What is the normal range for the motions?

*13. Using either loose bones or articulated models, mimic the motions of supination and pronation. Compare and describe the relative positions of the radius and ulna at the end-points of supination and pronation.

MYOLOGY OF THE ELBOW AND FOREARM

Use the following muscle sheets to aid in learning the origins, insertions, and innervations of the forearm muscles. For each of the muscles named, draw in the muscle on the sketch and complete the indicated information in the outline.

The following abbreviations apply throughout the muscle sheets:

O: Origin of muscle
I: Insertion of muscle
N: Innervation (both spinal level and peripheral nerve)
R: Relationship of muscle to axis of motion
A: Action of muscle

14. Biceps brachii

O: Short head—coracoid process of scapula;
   Long head—supraglenoid tubercle of scapula
I: Posterior aspect of radial tuberosity
N: Musculocutaneous n. (C-5, C-6)
R: Fibers run straight from superior O to inferior I; anterior to axis for shoulder flexion and extension (long head); anterior to axis for elbow flexion and extension; superior to and wraps around axis for supination and pronation
A:

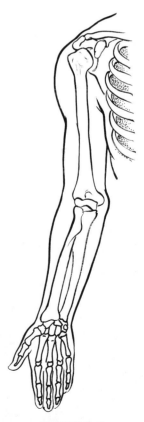

FIGURE 8–7

15. Supinator

    O: Lateral epicondyle of humerus; ulna, distal to radial notch; annular ligament and radial collateral ligament of elbow

    I: Dorsal and lateral surfaces of body of radius, distal to radial head

    N:

    R: Fibers run obliquely from superior O to inferior I; posterior to axis for pronation and supination

    A: Supination of the forearm

16. Triceps brachii

    O: Long head—
       Lateral head—
       Medial head—

    I: Posterior surface of proximal olecranon

    N: Radial n. (C-7, C-8)

    R: Fibers run obliquely, depending on head; shoulder (long head only)—posterior to axis for flexion and extension; medial to axis for abduction and adduction; elbow—posterior to axis for flexion and extension

    A: Long head—
       Lateral head—
       Medial head—

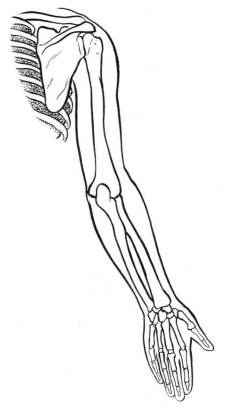

FIGURE 8–8

17. Brachialis

    O: Distal half of anterior surface of humerus

    I:

    N: Musculocutaneous n. (C-5, C-6)

    R:

    A: Flexion of the ulna on the humerus

18. Brachioradialis

    O:

    I: Lateral side of radial styloid

    N:

    R: Anterior to axis for flexion and extension; anterior or posterior to axis for pronation and supination, depending upon starting position of forearm

    A:

19. Pronator teres

    O: Medial epicondyle of humerus; common flexor tendon; and coronoid process

    I:

    N: Median n. (C-6, C-7)

    R:

    A:

20. Pronator quadratus

    O:

    I:

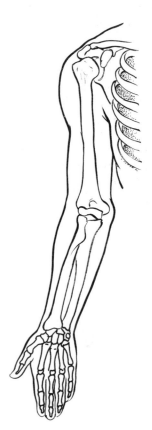

FIGURE 8–7

N:

R: Anterior to axis for pronation and supination

A: Pronation of the forearm

APPLICATIONS

21. What are the functional implications of an adhesion between the head of the radius and the annular ligament?

*22. A patient presents with weakness of elbow flexion. Without consulting a muscle-testing textbook, demonstrate how you would differentiate weakness in the biceps, brachialis, and brachioradialis by appropriately positioning the patient and the upper extremity to emphasize one muscle over the others.

*23. Position the subject's upper extremity to stretch the brachialis muscle without interference from a possibly tight biceps muscle. How did you confirm that your position was appropriate?

* 24. Position the subject's upper extremity to put the long head of the triceps on maximal stretch. How did you determine that the long head was actually on maximal stretch?

*25. Place the subject's upper extremity so that:

a. The biceps is at a position in which it produces its weakest contraction

b. The triceps is at a position in which it produces its weakest contraction

c. What principle are you applying in these two activities?

*26. If the radius and ulna were fused, what joints could a person use to turn the palm of the hand up enough to accept a coin without dropping it? Demonstrate your answer. What is the importance of this observation to accurate goniometric evaluation of forearm supination and pronation?

*27. Place your subject in a position so that contraction of the pectoralis major and anterior deltoid will extend the elbow.

28. How does the distal humerus act as a pulley for the triceps?

29. Diagram (using an end view or cross section of the radius) the mechanism by which the biceps brachii causes supination of the forearm.

*30. Demonstrate and describe the movement of the glenohumeral and humeroulnar joints that will allow the biceps to flex the elbow with strength through the largest possible range. What principle is being demonstrated in this activity?

31. Forearm supination and pronation may be limited by tightness or adhesions in which ligament(s)? Be sure to consider all relevant joints. Explain your answer.

32. Extension of the forearm at the elbow may be limited by tightness or adhesions in which ligament(s)? Be sure to consider all relevant joints. Explain your answer.

33. What muscle(s) could serve as a neutralizer or neutralizers for the biceps when you flex the forearm at the elbow with the forearm in pronation?

34. Assume that you would treat pain at the epicondyles of the elbow by resting the muscles attached to the epicondyle. How would your treatment of pain at the lateral epicondyle differ from treatment of pain at the medial epicondyle?

35. Describe how you would differentiate between limited motion in the humeroulnar joint and a biceps brachii that is too short.

ANSWERS TO ELBOW AND FOREARM

*1. Use your texts to identify the landmarks. Then have a faculty member confirm your palpations.

2. Check your text to confirm your information.

3. Check your text to confirm your information.

4. The purpose of the interosseous membrane is:
    a. To transfer force from the radius to the ulna, and through the ulna to the humerus.
    b. To provide stability for the radioulnar joints. The alignment of fibers from proximal on the radius to distal on the ulna allows for the efficient transfer of force from the radius to the ulna. Fibers oriented in other directions provide stability of the superior and inferior radioulnar joints.

5. To maintain the head of the radius in close contact with the ulna and to stabilize the head of the radius during supination and pronation.

6. The humeroulnar joint is part of a compound synovial joint with the humeroradial joint that allows approximately 135° to 145° of active flexion and 0° of extension. This motion occurs through the gliding of the ulna around the trochlea of the humerus. One degree of freedom is available.

    Humeroulnar Joint

    Type of joint—compound synovial joint, hinge joint.
    Type of motion that occurs at joint—flexion and extension by the humerus rolling within the olecranon or the olecranon rolling around the humerus.
    Amount of motion available at joint—135° to 145° of flexion and 0° of extension; one degree of freedom.

7. Humeroradial joint

    Type of joint—part of a compound synovial joint with the humeroulnar joint.
    Type of motion that occurs at joint—elbow flexion and extension through the gliding of the radial head around the capitulum of the humerus.
    Pivoting of the radial head on the capitulum is also required for pronation and supination to occur.

8. During flexion in an open kinematic chain, the concave surfaces of the radius and ulna glide anteriorly around the convex capitulum and trochlea of the humerus. During extension, the surfaces glide posteriorly.

*9. Elbow extension should have a hard end-feel because the olecranon process contacts the olecranon fossa at the end of the range. The end-feel for flexion is soft or springy because the forearm flexor musculature contacts the elbow flexor musculature at the end of the range of flexion.

10. Proximal radioulnar joint

Type of joint—synovial pivot joint.

Type of motion that occurs at joint—the radial head is contained within the annular ligament as it pivots on the capitulum of the humerus and the radial notch of the ulna; the resultant motion is pronation and supination of the forearm.

11. Distal radioulnar joint

Type of joint—synovial pivot joint.

Type of motion that occurs at joint—the distal radius glides around the distal aspect of the ulna, allowing pronation and supination.

12. Pronation and supination. Approximately 80° to 90° of each is present, though pronation is often slightly less than supination.

*13. Confirm your motions with a faculty member. Note that the proximal end of the radius rotates, but remains in the same position relative to the capitulum and proximal ulna, whereas the distal aspect of the radius rotates around the distal ulna, moving from the lateral aspect of the ulna in supination to the medial aspect in pronation.

14. Biceps brachii

O: Short head—coracoid process of scapula; Long head—supraglenoid tubercle of scapula
I: Posterior aspect of radial tuberosity
N: Musculocutaneous n. (C-5, C-6)
R: Fibers run straight from superior O to inferior I; anterior to axis for shoulder flexion and extension (long head); anterior to axis for elbow flexion and extension; superior to and wraps around axis for supination and pronation
A: Shoulder flexion (long head); elbow flexion; forearm supination

15. Supinator

O: Lateral epicondyle of humerus; ulna, distal to radial notch; annular ligament and radial collateral ligament of elbow
I: Dorsal and lateral surfaces of body of radius, distal to radial head
N: Radial n. (C-6)
R: Fibers run obliquely from superior O to inferior I; posterior to axis for pronation and supination
A: Supination of the forearm

16. Triceps brachii

O: Long head—infraglenoid tubercle of scapula; Lateral head—posterior humerus, proximal to groove for radial n.; Medial head—posterior surface humerus, distal aspect
I: Posterior surface of proximal olecranon
N: Radial n. (C-7, C-8)
R: Fibers run obliquely, depending on head; shoulder (long head only)—posterior to axis for flexion and extension; medial to axis for abduction and adduction; elbow—posterior to axis for flexion and extension
A: Long head—shoulder and elbow extension and shoulder adduction; Lateral and medial heads—elbow extension

17. Brachialis

O: Distal half of anterior surface of humerus
I: Coronoid process of ulna and ulnar tuberosity
N: Musculocutaneous n. (C-5, C-6)
R: Anterior to axis for flexion and extension
A: Flexion of the elbow

18. Brachioradialis

    O: Lateral supracondylar ridge of humerus

    I: Lateral side of radial styloid

    N: Radial n. (C-5, C-6)

    R: Anterior to axis for flexion and extension; anterior or posterior to axis for pronation and supination, depending upon starting position of forearm

    A: Elbow flexion; pronation from fully supinated position to neutral; supination from fully pronated position to neutral

19. Pronator teres

    O: Medial epicondyle of humerus; common flexor tendon; coronoid process of ulna

    I: Lateral aspect of middle of radial shaft

    N: Median n. (C-6, C-7)

    R: Anterior to axis for pronation and supination; anterior to axis for elbow flexion and extension

    A: Forearm pronation; elbow flexion (assists)

20. Pronator quadratus

    O: Anterior surface of distal ulna

    I: Anterior surface of distal radius

    N: Median n. (C-8, T-1)

    R: Anterior to axis for pronation and supination

    A: Pronation of the forearm

21. If the head of the radius is not free to rotate within the annular ligament, full pronation and supination cannot occur. Where the limitation would occur in the range of pronation and supination would depend on the position of the radius when the adhesion developed.

*22. Since the biceps brachii performs both supination and elbow flexion, use of this muscle can be detected by the combined motion. The brachioradialis can cause some forearm supination if the forearm is pronated and can cause some pronation if the forearm is supinated. Because of its insertion on the ulna, the brachialis performs no other action with elbow flexion. Using these characteristics, the examiner can determine which muscle is working by combining forearm position and palpation during elbow flexion.

    With the forearm supinated strongly, the biceps is the strongest flexor of the forearm. Its tendon can be palpated in the cubital fossa during elbow flexion.

    When the forearm is pronated and the elbow is flexed, the brachialis can be palpated on either side of the biceps brachii tendon. Since supination is being voluntarily inhibited, the brain will "choose" not to have the biceps brachii participate as much in elbow flexion.

    When the forearm is in neutral between pronation and supination and the elbow is flexed, the brachioradialis can easily be palpated along the radial aspect of the elbow and proximal forearm.

    A knowledge of the anatomy of the muscles of elbow flexion combined with palpation of those muscles can be used to determine which muscles are working most strongly to cause elbow flexion.

*23. Since the brachialis crosses only one joint and the biceps crosses two joints, placing the biceps so that it is slack over one joint would allow the brachialis to be stretched without interference from the tight biceps. Since the brachialis crosses only the elbow joint, it must be stretched over that joint. Therefore, the biceps would need to be put in a slack position over the shoulder joint. The position of choice for this activity would be shoulder flexion and elbow extension. Palpate the biceps tendon to be sure it remains slack while stretching the brachialis.

*24. The proximal attachment of the long head of the triceps is the infraglenoid tubercle of the scapula. The insertion is the olecranon process of the ulna. To maximally stretch this muscle, these two points need to be separated as much as possible. This is best done with maximum shoulder flexion combined with maximum elbow flexion.

*25. a. The weakest position of the biceps would be a combination of *either* extreme shoulder flexion, extreme elbow flexion, and extreme supination *or* extreme shoulder extension, extreme elbow extension, and extreme pronation. In these positions, voluntary activation of the biceps produces a relatively weak contraction.

   b. The weakest positions for the triceps would be similar—extreme shoulder flexion with extreme elbow flexion or extreme shoulder extension with extreme elbow extension. Supination and pronation would not affect the strength of the triceps. In either of the positions described, elbow extension and, to some extent, shoulder extension would be weakened.

   c. The principle being applied is active insufficiency of the muscle that is being asked to contract. The positions in which a muscle is weakest are extreme lengthening and extreme shortening. This is an application of the length-tension relationship.

*26. The shoulder and the carpal joints. By abducting and adducting the shoulder, a person can alter the position of the palm. The many carpal joints also allow some limited pronation and supination.

   For accurate goniometry, therefore, the shoulder must be controlled and the measurement should not include motion that occurs in the carpal joints. Both of these conditions can be met by aligning one arm of the goniometer with the humerus and the other with a line formed by the distal radius and ulna (across either the anterior or posterior surface of the distal forearm, proximal to the wrist).

*27. The pectoralis major can flex the humerus at the shoulder, as can the anterior deltoid. If the hand is stabilized while the elbow is flexed and the shoulder extended (as in sitting with the palm on the seat surface and elbow slightly flexed), contraction of the pectoralis major and anterior deltoid will cause shoulder flexion. With the hand stabilized, flexion of the humerus at the shoulder will cause extension of the elbow. Other muscles would also be active in the normal individual, such as the triceps. But if the triceps was not able to function, active elbow extension could still be accomplished in the manner described above, though it would not be particularly strong.

28. The distal humerus is angled anteriorly in comparison to the shaft of the humerus. This angulation causes the axis of motion of elbow flexion to be displaced anteriorly, which effectively increases the moment arm for the line of pull of the triceps.

29. The head of the radius is held next to the ulna by the annular ligament. During pronation and supination, the head of the radius rotates within this ligament. The biceps brachii inserts on the tuberosity of the radius. In pronation, the tuberosity is oriented more posteriorly, which wraps the tendon of the biceps around the radius (Figure 8-10). On contraction, the biceps causes the radius to "unwind" or supinate (Figure 8-9). It can be diagrammed as follows.

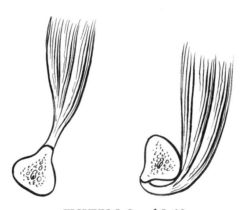

FIGURES 8–9 and 8–10

*30. By starting the motion with the humerus flexed moderately at the shoulder and the elbow extended, and then simultaneously extending the humerus at the shoulder and flexing the forearm at the elbow, the length-tension relationship of the biceps brachii is maintained in a stronger range. This will allow increased strength through the typically weaker end ranges of elbow motion. These motions will keep the biceps relatively stretched over one joint as it shortens over the other joint. This is an application of the length-tension relationship.

31. Since the interosseous membrane, the anterior radioulnar ligament, and the oblique cord all limit supination, abnormal limitation in any of them can cause decreased supination. The posterior radioulnar ligament limits pronation, so abnormal limitation of this ligament can cause decreased pronation. Excessive tightness of the annular ligament can also limit pronation and supination. It should be noted, however, that pronation is normally more limited by bony approximation than by ligamentous tightness.

32. Tightness of the anterior joint capsule, the anterior portions of the ulnar and radial collateral ligaments, and any of the muscles crossing the anterior surface of the elbow joint has the potential to decrease elbow extension. Tightness in these anterior structures would not allow the posterior motion of the radius and ulna over the distal portion of the humerus that is required for extension.

33. The two muscles that pronate the forearm are the pronator teres and the pronator quadratus. Either or both of these muscles could neutralize the supination component of the biceps brachii during elbow flexion.

34. You must first determine what muscles attach to each area. The medial epicondyle generally serves as an attachment for the wrist and finger flexors. The lateral epicondyle serves as an attachment for the wrist and finger extensors.

    Pain at the lateral epicondyle might be treated by resting the wrist and finger extensors. Remember that the wrist extensors are a strong synergist for the finger flexors. In fact, more extensor activity is probably generated by this synergy than primary use of the extensors. Therefore, finger and wrist flexion may also need to be limited. Pain at the medial epicondyle, on the other hand, would require rest of the wrist and finger flexors.

35. If the biceps brachii is tight, it will limit the amount of shoulder extension, elbow extension, and forearm pronation that is available. Unless the muscle is very tight, though, if the extremity is positioned in the extremes of two of those motions, the third motion will not be affected. Therefore, you would not expect a tight biceps brachii to limit elbow flexion when the shoulder is flexed and the forearm is supinated.

    If the humeroulnar joint is tight, however, shoulder and forearm position will have no effect on the motion available at that joint. So, to determine whether a tight biceps brachii or a tight joint is the problem, you would compare the amount of elbow extension with the shoulder flexed and the forearm supinated with the amount of elbow extension with the shoulder extended and the forearm pronated. If there is no difference in the amount of motion in the two positions, you would suspect that the joint is the limiting factor. If there are different amounts of elbow extension in the two positions, you would suspect that the biceps brachii was the limiting factor.

9 WRIST AND HAND

OSTEOLOGY AND ARTHROLOGY OF THE WRIST AND HAND

*1. Identify the following landmarks or structures on a laboratory partner.

Radial styloid
Ulnar styloid
Hook of hamate
Scaphoid (navicular)
Triquetrum
Capitate
Pisiform
Sesamoid bones of thumb (tendon of Add. Pol.)
Base, shaft, and head of each metacarpal
Base, shaft, and head of each phalanx
Joint line of MCP (metacarpophalangeal) and
   PIP (proximal interphalangeal) joints

Flexor retinaculum
Tendons:
   Flexor carpi ulnaris
   Flexor carpi radialis
   Extensor carpi radialis longus and brevis
   Extensor carpi ulnaris
   Interossei (palmar and dorsal)
   Flexor digitorum superficialis and profundus
   Extensor indicis
   Extensor digiti minimi
   Extensor digitorum

2. Complete the following outline in relation to the joints of the wrist and hand:

Wrist Joint (Radiocarpal Joint)

Bones involved

Type of joint

Name(s) of motion(s) at joint

Amount of motion available at joint

Midcarpal Joints

Bones involved

Type of joint

Name(s) of motion(s) at joint

Amount of motion available at joint

Carpometacarpal Joint of Thumb

Bones involved

Type of joint

Name(s) of motion(s) at joint

Carpometacarpal Joints of Fingers

Bones involved

Type of joint

Name(s) of motion(s) at joint

Metacarpophalangeal Joints

Bones involved

Type of joint

Name(s) of motion(s) at joint

Amount of motion available at joint

Interphalangeal Joints

Bones involved

Type of joint

Name(s) of motion(s) at joint

Amount of motion available at joint

NEUROLOGY OF THE WRIST AND HAND

3. Describe the peripheral nerve *sensory* distribution to the hand. Why are we asking you about the sensory distribution in the hand when we have not mentioned sensory considerations in any other area?

4. Describe the peripheral nerve *motor* distribution to the intrinsic muscles of the hand. What is the relationship of the innervation of the intrinsics and the extrinsics?

MYOLOGY OF THE WRIST AND HAND

Use of the following muscle sheets to aid in learning the origins, insertions, and innervations of muscles of the wrist and hand. For each of the muscles named, draw in the muscle on the sketch and complete the indicated information on the outlines.

    O: Origin of muscle

    I: Insertion of muscle

    N: Innervation (both spinal level and peripheral nerve)

    R: Relationship of muscle to the axis of motion

    A: Action of muscle

Muscles of the Wrist

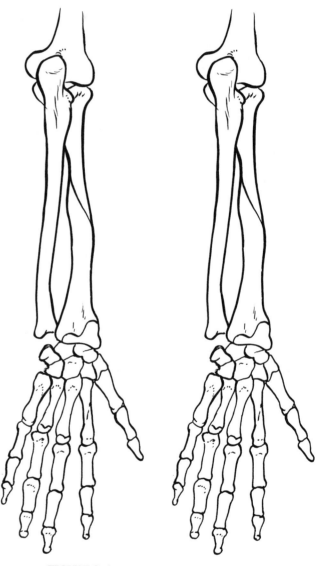

5. Extensor carpi radialis longus

    O:

    I: Dorsal surface, base of index metacarpal

    N:

    R: Posterior to axis for flexion and extension of wrist; radial to axis for abduction and adduction of wrist

    A: Wrist extension; wrist radial deviation (limited)

6. Extensor carpi radialis brevis

    O: Lateral epicondyle of humerus

    I:

    N: Radial n. (C-6, C-7)

    R:

    A: Wrist extension

7. Extensor carpi ulnaris

    O: Lateral epicondyle of humerus

    I: Ulnar side of base of fifth metacarpal

    N:

    R:

    A:

FIGURE 9–1   **FIGURE 9–1**

8. Flexor carpi ulnaris

   O:

   I:

  N: Ulnar n. (C-8, T-1)

  R: Palmar to axis for flexion and extension of wrist; ulnar to axis for abduction and adduction; anterior to axis for flexion and extension of elbow

  A:

9. Flexor carpi radialis

   O: Medial epicondyle of humerus

   I:

  N:

  R:

  A: Wrist flexion; wrist radial deviation; elbow flexion

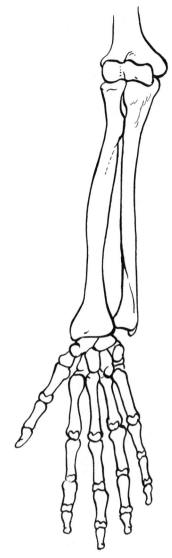

FIGURE 9–2

Extrinsic Muscles of the Hand

10. Extensor digitorum

    O:

    I:

    N:

    R: Dorsal to axes for flexion and extension of MCPs, IPs, and wrist; neutral to axes for abduction and adduction of wrist, MCPs, and IPs

    A: Wrist extension; MCP extension; IP extension

11. Extensor indicis

    O: Dorsal surface of ulna distal to thumb extensor

    I:

    N: Radial n. (C-6, C-7, C-8)

    R: Posterior to axes for flexion and extension of MCP and IP; neutral to axis for abduction and adduction of MCP; posterior to axis for flexion and extension of wrist

    A:

12. Extensor digiti minimi

    O: Lateral epicondyle of humerus

    I: Extensor mechanism of fifth digit

    N:

    R: Dorsal to axes for flexion and extension of MCP and IP; neutral to axis for abduction and adduction of MCP

    A:

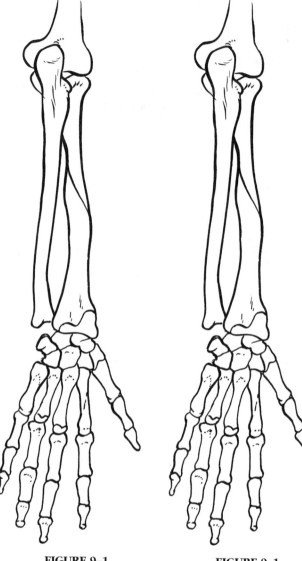

FIGURE 9–1   **FIGURE 9–1**

13. Extensor pollicis brevis

O: Distal third of dorsal surface of radius

I:

N: Radial n. (C-6, C-7)

R: Posterior to axis for MCP flexion and extension; dorsal to axis for wrist flexion and extension; radial to axis for wrist abduction and adduction

A:

14. Extensor pollicis longus

O:

I: Base of distal phalanx of thumb, dorsal surface

N: Radial n. (C-6, C-7, C-8)

R: Dorsal to axes for flexion and extension of wrist, MCP, IP; radial to axis for abduction and adduction of wrist; neutral to axis for abduction and adduction of thumb MCP

A:

15. Abductor pollicis longus

O: Dorsal surface of middle of both ulna and radius

I: Radial side of base of first metacarpal

N:

R:

A: Abduction of MC (metacarpal carpal) joint of thumb; radial deviation of wrist; flexion of wrist

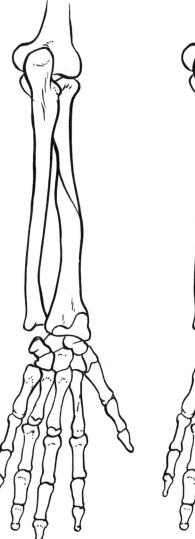
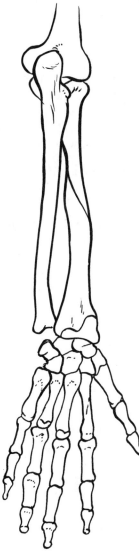

FIGURE 9–1 **FIGURE 9–1**

16. Flexor digitorum superficialis

   O:

    I:

   N:

   R: Neutral to axes for abduction and adduction of wrist and MCP; palmar to axes for flexion and extension of wrist, MCPs, and PIPs

   A: PIP flexion of digits 2–5; MCP flexion of digits 2–5; wrist flexion

17. Flexor digitorum profundus

   O:

    I:

   N: Digits 2, 3—median n. (C-8, T-1); digits 4, 5—ulnar n. (C-8, T-1)

   R: Palmar to axes for wrist, MCP, PIP, DIP (distal interphalangeal) flexion and extension; neutral to axis for abduction and adduction of wrist and MCP

   A:

18. Flexor pollicis longus

   O:

    I:

   N: Median n. (C-8, T-1)

   R:

   A: Flexion of thumb MCP; flexion of thumb IP; wrist flexion; radial deviation of wrist (minimal)

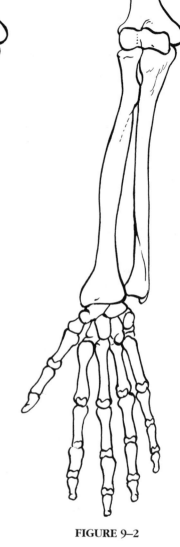
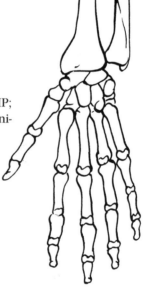

FIGURE 9–2   **FIGURE 9–2**

Intrinsic Muscles of the Hand

19. Opponens pollicis

    O:

    I: Radial side of length of first metacarpal

    N:

    R: Medial to axis for flexion and extension of MC joint of thumb; palmar to axis for abduction and adduction of MC joint; ulnar to axis for rotation of MC joint

    A:

20. Opponens digiti minimi

    O:

    I: Ulnar side of fifth metacarpal

    N: Ulnar n. (C-8, T-1)

    R: Radial to axis for opposition of fifth metacarpal joint

    A:

21. Abductor digiti minimi

    O: Pisiform; tendon of flexor carpi ulnaris

    I:

    N: Ulnar n. (C-8)

    R:

    A: MCP ulnar deviation; MCP flexion

22. Dorsal interossei

    O:

    I:

    N: Ulnar n. (C-8, T-1)

    R: Palmar to axis for flexion and extension of MCP; radial to axis for abduction and adduction of index and long fingers; ulnar to axis for abduction and adduction of long and ring fingers

    A:

23. Adductor pollicis

    O:

    I: Base of proximal phalanx of thumb

    N: Ulnar n. (C-8, T-1)

    R:

    A:

24. Abductor pollicis brevis

    O: Scaphoid; trapezium; transverse carpal ligament

    I:

    N: Median n. (C-6, C-7)

    R: Radial to axis for abduction and adduction of MCP; radial to axis for abduction and adduction of MC joint

    A:

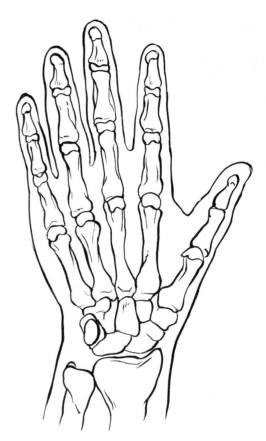

FIGURE 9–3

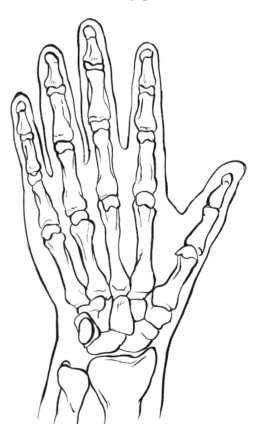

FIGURE 9–3

25. Flexor pollicis brevis

   O:

    I: Base of proximal phalanx, palmar surface

   N: Radial portion—median n. (C-6, C-7); Ulnar portion—ulnar n. (C-8, T-1)

   R: Palmar to axes for flexion of MCP and IP of thumb

   A: Thumb MCP and IP flexion

26. Palmar interossei

   O:

    I:

   N: Ulnar n. (C-8, T-1)

   R: Palmar to axis for MCP flexion and extension; index—ulnar to axis for abduction and adduction of MCP; ring and little—radial to axis for abduction and adduction of MCP; dorsal to axes for flexion and extension of IP joints

   A:

27. Lumbricals

   O:

    I: Radial aspect of extensor mechanism of each finger at the level of the MCP joint

   N: First and second lumbricals—median n. (C-6, C-7); Third and fourth lumbricals—ulnar n. (C-8)

   R:

   A:

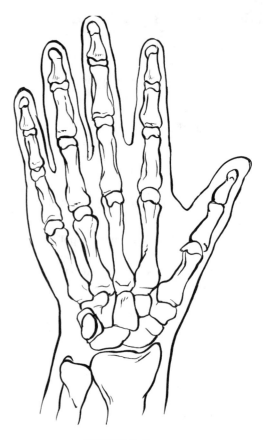

FIGURE 9–3

APPLICATIONS

28. What is the purpose of the sheaths surrounding the flexor tendons?

*29. Use a string to represent your flexor digitorum profundus. Tape the string to the pad of a fingertip. Pull on the string to represent a contraction of the long flexor.

   a. What happens to the string when you pull it and allow your finger to flex?

   b. What keeps this from happening with the "real" tendons in your finger?

   c. What would happen if the restraining structures in b were not intact?

*30. Review the definition of *synergy* and demonstrate two synergies that normally occur when using the hand.

31. Label the indicated items on the diagram of the extensor mechanism below.

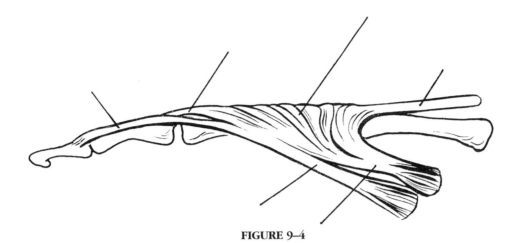

FIGURE 9–4

*32. Demonstrate the "intrinsic position" (the position the fingers assume when the lumbricals and interossei are contracting simultaneously or are shortened).

*33. In what position would you place the fingers in order to stretch the intrinsic muscles? Perform the motion on yourself and feel for any tightness.

*34. What is the functional significance of loss of the median nerve at the wrist level? Remember to consider both sensory and motor problems that might occur. To simulate the sensory deficit, get a pair of surgical gloves. Turn one inside out. Cut the small and ring fingers off the gloves. Put both gloves on one hand. Now put your gloved hand in your pocket or pocketbook and find a quarter or some other small object that you know is there. Can you tell a quarter from a nickel without looking? Describe how you chose to identify the coins or objects. Don't forget to simulate the lack of median-innervated musculature.

*35. What is the functional significance of loss of the ulnar nerve at the wrist level? Remember to consider both sensory and motor problems that might occur. Again, use surgical gloves to simulate the loss of sensation. Alter a new set of gloves to cover the area of skin innervated by the ulnar nerve. Don't forget to simulate the lack of ulnar-innervated musculature.

36. Based on activities 34 and 35, do you think a median or an ulnar nerve lesion at the wrist level would be more debilitating in functional terms? Give your rationale.

37. What symptoms would you expect to see with edema in the carpal tunnel and why?

*38. Have a laboratory partner firmly grip two of your fingers. Now, have your partner do the same thing with her wrist in *extreme* flexion. Repeat this one more time with *extreme* wrist extension. Which was strongest, which was weakest, and why?

*39. What is a major benefit of having the extrinsic finger flexors and extensors crossing multiple joints?

*40. a. What would be the effect of scarring in the flexor sheath of a single finger?

   b. What is the effect of this limitation on making a fist? Give a rationale.

*41. Go to your texts and review the musculotendinous anatomy of the flexor digitorum profundus and superficialis.

    a. What is a primary difference in the structure of the two muscles?

    b. With the back of your right hand on a table, immobilize your right index, long, and small fingers in complete MCP, PIP, and DIP extension while you flex your ring finger MCP with your left hand. Actively flex your right ring finger PIP and DIP in this position. What happened at the PIP? Why? What happened at the DIP? Why?

    c. Relate this finding to muscle testing to isolate the superficialis from the profundus.

42. How would you differentiate between a tight tendon (the musculotendinous unit not being long enough) and a stiff PIP joint? Demonstrate the test(s) that you would perform on a partner and indicate what muscles you would be concerned about.

43. A patient cut her profundus tendon to the ring finger and a surgeon repaired it. The physician told you to keep the PIP joint mobile, but put little or no stress over the repair (in other words, you cannot pull on the tendon). How could this task be accomplished?

ANSWERS TO WRIST AND HAND

*1. Check your text to find these items and then have a faculty member confirm your information.

2. **Wrist Joint (Radiocarpal Joint)**

    Bones involved—radius, radioulnar disc, triquetrum, lunate, and scaphoid (navicular)

    Type of joint—synovial, condyloid

    Names of motions at joint—flexion and extension, and radial and ulnar deviation

    Amount of motion available at joint—the various components of the wrist joint are not able to be measured separately for their contributions to wrist motion. Total wrist motion is approximately 80° to 90° of flexion, 75° to 85° of extension, 15° of radial deviation, and 45° of ulnar deviation.

    Midcarpal Joint

    Bones involved—scaphoid, lunate, and triquetrum proximally; trapezium, trapezoid, capitate, and hamate distally

    Type of joint—complex of synovial plane joints

    Names of motions at joints—flexion and extension, and radial and ulnar deviation

    Amount of motion available at joints (see comments for radiocarpal joint)

    Carpometacarpal Joint of Thumb

    Bones involved—trapezium and first (or thumb) metacarpal

    Type of joint—synovial, saddle

    Names of motions at joint—flexion and extension, abduction and adduction, rotation, opposition

Carpometacarpal Joints of Fingers

Bones involved—distal carpal row and bases of second (or index finger) through fifth (or small finger) metacarpals

Type of joint—synovial, plane

Name of motions at joint—flexion and extension

Metacarpophalangeal Joints

Bones involved—metacarpal and proximal phalanx of each finger

Type of joint—synovial, condyloid

Names of motions at joint—flexion and extension, radial and ulnar deviation

Amount of motion available at joint—approximately 85° to 105° of flexion, 20° to 30° of extension, and 20° to 25° each of radial and ulnar deviation

Interphalangeal Joints

Bones involved—adjacent phalanges for each finger. Note that the index, long, ring, and small fingers each have a proximal and a distal interphalangeal joint, while the thumb has only one interphalangeal joint.

Type of joint—synovial, hinge

Name of motion at joint—flexion and extension

Amount of motion available at joint—proximal interphalangeal joints (PIPs) have from 100° to 110° of flexion and typically extend to neutral without hyperextension. Distal interphalangeal joints (DIPs) typically have 80° to 90° of flexion and extend to neutral or slightly beyond.

3. The median nerve provides sensation for the thenar half of the palm and the palmar surface of the thumb, index, long, and half of the ring finger. The ulnar nerve innervates the rest of the palmar surface of the hand. The radial nerve innervates the dorsum of the hand, though there is a great deal of overlap with the median and ulnar nerves on the dorsum of the hand.

   The hand is the primary organ that interacts with the environment through touch. Sensation is needed for protection and information gathering. Sensory information is transmitted along the sensory components of the peripheral nerves.

4. The lumbricals are innervated by the same nerve that innervates the flexor digitorum profundus muscle to which the lumbrical is attached (i.e., lumbricals 1 and 2 are innervated by the median nerve and lumbricals 3 and 4 are innervated by the ulnar nerve). All of the interossei are innervated by the ulnar nerve. The thenar muscles, with the exception of the adductor pollicis and the deep head of the flexor pollicis brevis, which are innervated by the ulnar nerve, are innervated by the median nerve.

5. Extensor carpi radialis longus

   O: Distal part of lateral supracondylar ridge

   I: Dorsal surface, base of index metacarpal

   N: Radial n. (C-6, C-7)

   R: Posterior to axis for flexion and extension of wrist; radial to axis for abduction and adduction of wrist

   A: Wrist extension; wrist radial deviation (limited)

6. Extensor carpi radialis brevis

   O: Lateral epicondyle of humerus

   I: Dorsal surface, base of long metacarpal

   N: Radial n. (C-6, C-7)

   R: Posterior to axis for flexion and extension of wrist; neutral to axis for abduction and adduction of wrist

   A: Wrist extension

7. Extensor carpi ulnaris

   O: Lateral epicondyle of humerus

   I: Ulnar side of base of fifth metacarpal

   N: Radial n. (C-6, C-7, C-8)

   R: Posterior to axis for flexion and extension of wrist; ulnar to axis for abduction and adduction of wrist

   A: Wrist extension; wrist ulnar deviation

8. Flexor carpi ulnaris

   O: Medial epicondyle of humerus; proximal dorsal surface of ulna

   I: Pisiform; base of fifth metacarpal

  N: Ulnar n. (C-8, T-1)

  R: Palmar to axis for flexion and extension of wrist; ulnar to axis for abduction and adduction of wrist; anterior to axis for flexion and extension of elbow

  A: Wrist flexion; wrist ulnar deviation; elbow flexion

9. Flexor carpi radialis

   O: Medial epicondyle of humerus

   I: Base of index metacarpal, palmar surface

  N: Median n. (C-6, C-7)

  R: Palmar to axis for flexion and extension of wrist; radial to axis for abduction and adduction; anterior to axis for flexion and extension of elbow

  A: Wrist flexion; wrist radial deviation; elbow flexion

Extrinsic Muscles of the Hand

10. Extensor digitorum

   O: Lateral epicondyle of humerus

   I: Four tendons, one to extensor mechanism of each finger

  N: Radial n. (C-6, C-7, C-8)

  R: Dorsal to axes for flexion and extension of MCPs, IPs, and wrist; neutral to axis for abduction and adduction of wrist, MCPs, and IPs

  A: Wrist extension; MCP extension; IP extension

11. Extensor indicis

   O: Dorsal surface of ulna distal to thumb extensor

   I: Ulnar aspect of index extensor mechanism

  N: Radial n. (C-6, C-7, C-8)

  R: Posterior to axes for flexion and extension of MCP and IP; neutral to axis for abduction and adduction of MCP; posterior to axis for flexion and extension of wrist

  A: MCP extension; IP extension; wrist extension

12. Extensor digiti minimi

   O: Lateral epicondyle of humerus

   I: Extensor mechanism of fifth digit

  N: Radial n. (C-6, C-7, C-8)

  R: Dorsal to axes for flexion and extension of MCP and IP; neutral to axis for abduction and adduction of MCP

  A: MCP extension; IP extension; wrist extension

13. Extensor pollicis brevis

   O: Distal third of dorsal surface of radius

   I: Base of first phalanx of thumb, dorsal surface

  N: Radial n. (C-6, C-7)

  R: Posterior to axis for MCP flexion and extension; dorsal to axis for wrist flexion and extension; radial to axis for wrist abduction and adduction

  A: Wrist extension; wrist radial deviation; MCP extension of thumb

14. Extensor pollicis longus

    O: Lateral part of middle third of body of ulna, dorsal surface
    I: Base of distal phalanx of thumb, dorsal surface
    N: Radial n. (C-6, C-7, C-8)
    R: Dorsal to axes for flexion and extension of wrist, MCP, IP; radial to axis for abduction and adduction of wrist; neutral to axis for abduction and adduction of thumb MCP
    A: Wrist extension; wrist radial deviation; thumb MCP and IP extension

15. Abductor pollicis longus

    O: Dorsal surface of middle of both ulna and radius
    I: Radial side of base of first metacarpal
    N: Radial n. (C-6, C-7)
    R: Palmar to axes for thumb abduction and wrist flexion; radial to axis for abduction and adduction of wrist
    A: Abduction of MC joint of thumb; wrist radial deviation; wrist flexion

16. Flexor digitorum superficialis

    O: Medial epicondyle of humerus; coronoid process; palmar surface of mid-third of radius
    I: Tendons divide to insert on radial and ulnar aspects of volar surface of middle phalanges of digits 2–5
    N: Median n. (C-7, C-8, T-1)
    R: Neutral to axes for abduction and adduction of wrist and MCP; palmar to axes for flexion and extension of wrist, MCPs, and PIPs
    A: PIP flexion of digits 2–5; MCP flexion of digits 2–5; wrist flexion

17. Flexor digitorum profundus

    O: Palmar surface of proximal three-quarters of ulna
    I: Palmar surface of base of distal phalanges of digits 2–5
    N: Digits 2, 3—median n. (C-8, T-1); digits 4, 5—ulnar n. (C-8, T-1)
    R: Palmar to axes for wrist, MCP, PIP, DIP flexion and extension; neutral to axes for abduction and adduction of wrist and MCP
    A: Wrist flexion; MCP flexion; PIP flexion; DIP flexion

18. Flexor pollicis longus

    O: Palmar surface of middle third of radius; coronoid process of ulna
    I: Palmar surface of base of distal phalanx of thumb
    N: Median n. (C-8, T-1)
    R: Palmar to axis of flexion and extension of wrist; radial to axis of abduction and adduction of wrist; palmar to axes of flexion and extension of MCP and IP of thumb
    A: Flexion of thumb MCP; flexion of thumb IP; wrist flexion; radial deviation of wrist (minimal)

Intrinsic Muscles of the Hand

19. Opponens pollicis

    O: Trapezium; flexor retinaculum
    I: Radial side of length of first metacarpal
    N: Median n. (C-6, C-7)
    R: Medial to axis for flexion and extension of MC joint of thumb; palmar to axis for abduction and adduction of MC joint; ulnar to axis for rotation of MC joint
    A: MC opposition (flexion, abduction, rotation)

20. Opponens digiti minimi

    O: Hook of hamate; flexor retinaculum
    I: Ulnar side of fifth metacarpal
    N: Ulnar n. (C-8, T-1)
    R: Radial to axis for opposition of fifth MC joint
    A: Opposition of MC joint of little finger

21. Abductor digiti minimi

    O: Pisiform; tendon of flexor carpi ulnaris
    I: Ulnar side of first phalanx of fifth finger; extensor mechanism
    N: Ulnar n. (C-8)
    R: Ulnar to axis for abduction and adduction of MCP; palmar to axis for flexion and extension of MCP
    A: MCP ulnar deviation; MCP flexion

22. Dorsal interossei

    O: Adjacent sides of metacarpals
    I: Extensor mechanism (extensor hood) and base of proximal phalanges of index, long, and ring fingers: index—radial side; long—both sides; ring—ulnar side
    N: Ulnar n. (C-8, T-1)
    R: Palmar to axis for flexion and extension of MCP; radial to axis for abduction and adduction of index and long fingers; ulnar to axis for abduction and adduction of long and ring fingers; dorsal to axes for flexion and extension of IP joints
    A: MCP flexion; MCP deviation: index—radial; long—both; ring—ulnar; IP extension

23. Adductor pollicis

    O: Capitate and bases of index and long metacarpals; shaft of long metacarpal, palmar surface
    I: Base of proximal phalanx of thumb
    N: Ulnar n. (C-8, T-1)
    R: MCP—volar to axis for flexion and extension; MC—ulnar to axis for abduction and adduction
    A: MC adduction; MCP flexion

24. Abductor pollicis brevis

    O: Scaphoid; trapezium; transverse carpal ligament
    I: Radial side of base of first phalanx of thumb
    N: Median n. (C-6, C-7)
    R: Radial to axis for abduction and adduction of MCP; radial to axis for abduction and adduction of MC joint
    A: MC and MCP abduction

25. Flexor pollicis brevis

    O: Flexor retinaculum; trapezium; ulnar border of first metacarpal
    I: Base of proximal phalanx, palmar surface
    N: Radial portion—median n. (C-6, C-7); Ulnar portion—ulnar n. (C-8, T-1)
    R: Palmar to axes for flexion of MCP and IP of thumb
    A: Thumb MCP and IP flexion

26. Palmar interossei

    O: Palmar surface of length of index, ring, and little metacarpal
    I: Side of base of proximal phalanx of corresponding finger: index—ulnar side; ring and little—radial side; extensor expansion of each digit
    N: Ulnar n. (C-8, T-1)
    R: Palmar to axis for MCP flexion and extension; index—ulnar to axis for abduction and adduction of MCP; ring and little—radial to axis for abduction and adduction of MCP; dorsal to axes for flexion and extension of IP joints
    A: MCP flexion; MCP deviation: index—ulnar; ring—radial; small—radial; IP extension

27. Lumbricals

    O: Tendons of flexor digitorum profundus of each finger
    I: Radial aspect of extensor mechanism of each finger at the level of the MCP joint
    N: First and second lumbricals—Median n. (C-6, C-7); Third and fourth lumbricals—Ulnar n. (C-8)
    R: Palmar to axis for MCP flexion and extension; dorsal to axes for IP flexion and extension
    A: MCP flexion; IP extension

28. To decrease resistance of friction so that the tendons may glide easily.

* 29. a. The string pulls away from your phalanges and "bows" across the finger and palm.
       b. The flexor retinaculum and the annular ligaments.
       c. The annular ligaments are designed to hold the tendons that pass under them close to the bone. If they were not there, the tendons would be able to pull away from the bone (bowstringing). The shortest distance between two points is a straight line (as you saw in a above). If the flexor tendons were not held tightly to the phalanges, when the fingers were flexed in a fist, the tendons would attempt to pass in a straight line from their insertion to the palm, causing the skin to "web." The grip strength would be greatly compromised since so much of the muscle's force would be used to shorten the muscle belly.

* 30. One definition of synergy is muscles that work together for a common goal by assisting each other (biceps and brachialis), stabilizing for each other (scapular muscles for glenohumeral motion), or neutralizing unwanted motions (rotator cuff and deltoid).
    Grip or finger flexion is usually accompanied with wrist extension (stabilizing or neutralizing). Finger extension, conversely, is usually accompanied by wrist flexion (stabilizing or neutralizing). Flexor digitorum superficialis and profundus work together to produce strong flexion of the PIP joints.

31. Here is a labeled diagram of the extensor mechanism.

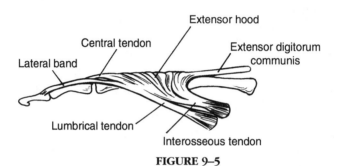

FIGURE 9–5

* 32. MCP flexion and IP extension comprise the shortened position of the intrinsic musculature.

* 33. MCP extension and IP flexion.

* 34. Loss of the median nerve at the wrist results in a loss of sensation over the median nerve distribution of the hand and loss of muscle function of the abductor pollicis brevis, opponens pollicis, part of flexor pollicis brevis, and first two lumbricals. Functionally, this would not allow one to position the thumb out of the plane of the palm, and opposition would be almost impossible. This motor deficit severely hampers the manipulative ability of the hand. The sensory loss is a major handicap because we depend so heavily on sensory input in the function of the hand. The manipulative aspects of the hand are the thumb, index, and long finger pads, and all of these surfaces are innervated by the median nerve.

* 35. Loss of the ulnar nerve at the wrist would result in a loss of sensation over the ulnar nerve distribution and loss of muscle function of the adductor pollicis, part of the flexor pollicis brevis, the interossei, and the two ulnar lumbricals. The weakness involved with ulnar nerve problems interferes with the ability to open or close the fingers in a broad arc. Instead of creating a coordinated opening that allows one to grasp a wide object, the fingers curl into the palm, pushing objects out of the palm. Curling the fingers into the palm means that all DIP and PIP flexion is completed first, and it is followed by MCP flexion. In the normal grasp, there is coordinated and simultaneous MCP, PIP, and DIP flexion. Try to pick up a drink can by first flexing your PIPs and DIPs and then flexing your MCPs.
    The functional significance of the sensory loss is that the ulnar aspect of the hand often comes into contact with the environment (resting on surfaces). Without sensation, an individual may not know whether the environment is safe (a tabletop) or hostile (a stove top).

36. There is no correct answer to this. With a median nerve loss, there is sensory loss to the finger and thumb

pads primarily used for interacting with the environment, and inability to lift the thumb from the plane of the palm, eliminating fine prehension. With an ulnar nerve loss, there is a sensory deficit over the ulnar aspect of the hand, and the person is able only to curl and uncurl the fingers (movement in a wide arc is not possible). See item 35 for a description of curling of the fingers.

Which injury is worse is debatable, but both significantly affect function. Generally, however, patients seem to have more limited function with a median nerve injury than with an ulnar nerve injury.

37. Edema would increase the pressure in the carpal tunnel. The structure in the tunnel most sensitive to increased pressure is the median nerve. The symptoms would be those of entrapment (interference with nerve transmission). The first symptoms are usually sensory disturbances in the median distribution of the hand. If the pressure continues, muscle weakness in the median innervated intrinsic musculature can result.

*38. Typically, the strongest grip position is the position that your partner chose without any instructions from the activity. The strongest position for finger flexion is usually mild wrist extension. The positions of extreme wrist flexion or extension usually create weaker grip strength because of a less than optimal length-tension relationship.

*39. By crossing many joints, the wrist and hand can have much finer control of the length-tension relationship of the extrinsic musculature. When one joint needs to be in a certain position for a specific activity, there are still several other joints that can be adjusted to maintain an optimal length-tension relationship.

Since the extrinsic muscles of the hand are multijoint muscles, they are highly sensitive to active and passive insufficiency. In extreme wrist flexion with active finger flexion, the finger flexors are actively insufficient and the finger extensors are often passively insufficient. In extreme wrist extension with finger extension, the finger flexors are often passively insufficient and the finger extensors are actively insufficient. The strongest position for finger flexion is usually mild wrist extension and the strongest position for finger extension is mild wrist flexion.

*40. Scarring in the flexor sheath acts as a tether and limits gliding of the tendon within the sheath. Depending where the tendon and sheath are adherent, flexion, extension, or both can be limited.
    a. Making a fist would be limited.
    b. The flexor digitorum profundus muscle belly tends to pull on all fingers simultaneously. Adhesions of the profundus in one finger, therefore, could limit excursion of the other fingers, though to a lesser degree. The flexor digitorum superficialis, on the other hand, has much more independence of finger function than the profundus. Scarring of a superficialis tendon in one finger would probably not have much of an effect on the other fingers.

*41. a. The profundus has one muscle belly with four interdependent tendons. The superficialis has muscle bellies that are more separated and more independent.
    b. Most people cannot flex the DIP joint in this position. The PIP flexes readily. This position effectively immobilizes the profundus tendon of all fingers except the ring finger. This could simulate scarring in the flexor sheath of a finger. Since the profundus has one muscle belly to activate four tendons, the limitation of one or more tendons limits the motion of all of the tendons.
    c. Using the position described in this exercise, you can effectively eliminate the contribution of the profundus muscle to flexion of any finger. This allows you to assess the strength of the superficialis. Free flexion of the fingers is the result of both profundus and superficialis function.

42. To differentiate between a tight tendon and a stiff joint, you must determine whether or not the positions of other joints affected by the tendon you are testing affects the motion of the joint you are testing. For instance, if you are trying to decide whether or not a PIP joint is stiff or the superficialis is tight, you would put the superficialis on slack (wrist and MCP flexion) and see if that affects the tightness of the PIP joint. If the joint is stiff, no change will occur in the joint as you change the position of the wrist and MCP joints. If, however, the superficialis is tight, as you flex the wrist and MCP, the PIP will be able to extend more. The same principle applies to the profundus at the DIP joint. Both the profundus and the superficialis could affect the motion of the PIP joint. You would be able to determine whether the profundus or the superficialis was tight by observing what happens at the DIP joint with wrist and MCP motion.

43. To extend the PIP joint and put minimal stress on the profundus tendon, all of the joints that the profundus crosses other than the PIP joint need to be positioned to put the profundus on slack. In that position, you can move the PIP joint into *some* extension without stressing the tendon. Therefore, the wrist, MCP, and DIP joints would all be in maximal flexion so that you could take the PIP joint into some extension. How would you apply this principle to keep the MCP joint mobile?

10 TEMPOROMANDIBULAR JOINT

OSTEOLOGY OF THE TEMPOROMANDIBULAR JOINT

*1. Palpate the following structures on a laboratory partner and label them on Figure 10-1.

Mandible
  Condyle (from lateral aspect of face)
  Condyle (from external auditory meatus)
  Coronoid process
  Angle
  Ramus
  Body
Zygomatic arch
Hyoid bone

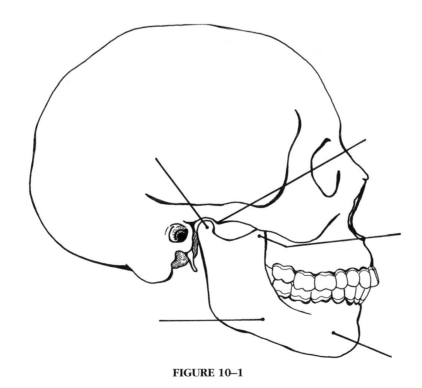

FIGURE 10–1

*2. Observe your partner for facial symmetry. Are the eyes and ears level? Are the nose and mouth in the center of the face? Is the mandible centered? Observe at least three people. Did you find symmetry or asymmetry more often?

ARTHROLOGY OF THE TEMPOROMANDIBULAR JOINT

*3. The following diagrams demonstrate the two components of joint motion during mouth opening. The condyle first rotates in the mandibular fossa (Figure 10–2A and B) and then glides downward and forward over the articular eminence (Figure 10–2B and C). Using a skull and a mandible, demonstrate both of these motions.

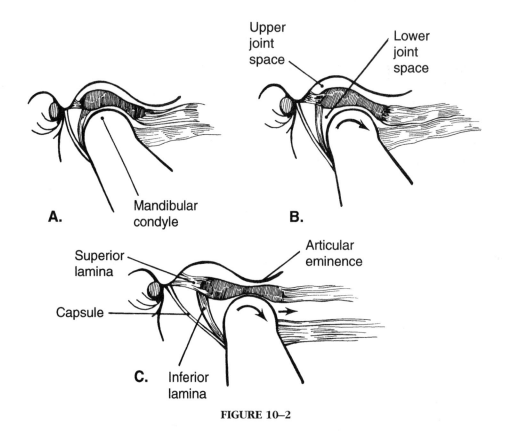

FIGURE 10–2

*4. On a laboratory partner, palpate the temporomandibular joint (TMJ) on mouth opening and mouth closing. Two methods of palpation are: (1) place your fingers lightly just anterior to the ear lobes and request that the person open and close the mouth gently, and (2) place your little finger inside the external auditory meatus and palpate the anterior aspect of the canal as the mouth opens and closes. Can you feel when rotation and translation occur in the range of motion? Did the joints move symmetrically? Did you feel any popping or clicking?

5. If you were to observe someone with a normal TMJ opening and closing his mouth, would you expect to see any lateral deviation?

6. The mandible has two articulations, one at each condyle. What are the implications of this arrangement on independent joint motion?

7. A disc covers the condyle like a sock. Consult texts and describe the attachments of the disc to the condyle and to other structures.

8. Describe how the disc moves during normal mouth opening and closing.

*9. On at least three laboratory partners, observe normal jaw movement and determine how you might measure it. The movements you want to observe and measure are mouth opening and closing, lateral deviation to each side, protrusion (jutting the jaw forward), and retrusion (sliding the jaw backward). Describe your measurement technique. Measure the laboratory partners using the methods you develop. What ranges of motion did you observe?

*10. On at least three laboratory partners, observe for lateral deviation of the mandible during mouth opening and closing. Choose a landmark (the spaces between the front teeth are often convenient) and ask the subject to open and close his mouth slowly. Do the two points you are observing keep the same relation throughout the motion? If they do not, what pattern does the deviation follow (e.g., a right or left C-curve, an S-curve)?

MYOLOGY OF THE TEMPOROMANDIBULAR JOINT

*11. Palpate the following muscles on a laboratory partner:

Masseter	Suprahyoid muscles
Temporalis	Scalenes (anterior, middle)
Infrahyoid muscles	Sternocleidomastoid

Use the following muscle sheets to aid in learning the origins, insertions, and innervations of the muscles of the TMJ. For each of the muscles described, find its placement on a skull.

O: Origin of muscle
I: Insertion of muscle
N: Innervation
R: Relationship of muscle to axis of motion
A: Action of muscle

12. Masseter

  O: Zygomatic arch
  I: Coronoid process, ramus, and angle of
     mandible
  N: Trigeminal n.—cranial n. V
  R: Anterior to axis for elevation and depression
  A: Elevates mandible

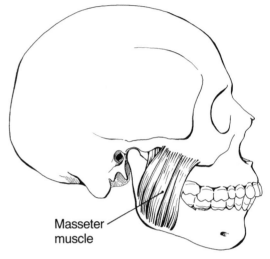

Masseter muscle

FIGURE 10–3

13. Temporalis

  O: Temporal fossa and fascia
  I: Coronoid process and anterior border of ramus
     of mandible
  N: Trigeminal n.—cranial n. V
  R: Anterior to axis for elevation and depression
  A: Elevates and retracts mandible

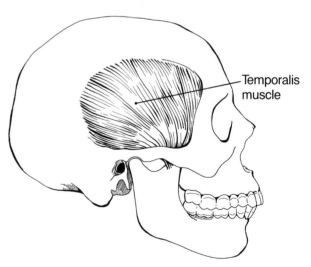

Temporalis muscle

FIGURE 10–4

14. Medial pterygoid

   O: Medial surface of lateral pterygoid plate
   I: Medial surface of ramus and angle of mandible
   N: Trigeminal n.—cranial n. V
   R: Translatory motion, axis irrelevant; muscle in line with motion
   A: Unilateral action: protrusion and lateral deviation to the opposite side
   Bilateral action: elevation of mandible

15. Lateral pterygoid

   O: Sphenoid and lateral surface of lateral pterygoid plate
   I: Front of condyle of mandible, anterior portion of the disc, and capsule of joint
   N: Trigeminal n.—cranial nerve V
   R: Translatory motion, axis irrelevant; muscle in line with motion
   A: Unilateral action: protrusion and deviation to opposite side
   Bilateral action: lower portion active during mandibular depression; superior portion active during mandibular elevation

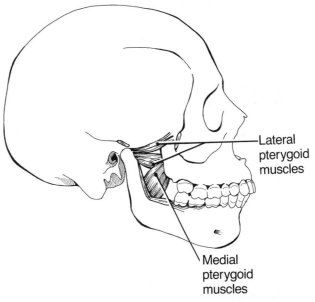

Lateral pterygoid muscles

Medial pterygoid muscles

FIGURE 10–5

16. Digastric

   O: Mastoid
   I: Through pulley attached to hyoid to posterior aspect of center of mandible
   N: Facial n.—cranial n. VII
   R: Posterior to axis for elevation and depression
   A: Depresses the mandible or elevates the hyoid

   See also:

   All neck musculature
   Sternocleidomastoid
   Scalenes (anterior, posterior, middle)

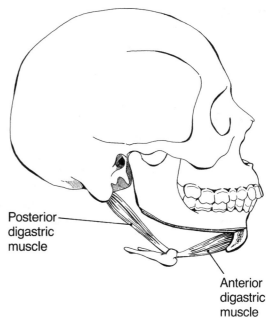

Posterior digastric muscle

Anterior digastric muscle

FIGURE 10–6

17. Describe the forces that control the motion of the disc during normal mouth opening and closing. Refer to your answer to item 8 in completing this item.

APPLICATIONS

*18. If the disc dislocates posteriorly, what motion of the condyle would be limited? If the disk dislocates anteriorly, what motion of the condyle would be limited? Explain why these limitations occur. Use a skull to demonstrate these situations.

*19. What would be the effect of an injury or obstruction that allowed only the rotation component of joint motion during mouth opening to occur in the left temporomandibular joint (TMJ) while the right TMJ could both rotate and glide. Assume that the right TMJ has normal motion. What would you see on mouth opening and closing? Re-create these problems with a skull and mandible.

*20. Describe the jaw motion on opening and closing that you would expect to see in the following two people:

Julia has a tight joint capsule of the left TMJ that limits translation.

Louis has an anteriorly dislocated left disc that reduces on mouth opening and dislocates on mouth closing.

*21. Sit with erect posture (normal primary and secondary curves). In that position, gently tap your teeth together and feel where they touch. Now put your chin on your chest and tap your teeth together. Next, look at the ceiling and tap your teeth together. Finally, tap your teeth together while you are in a forward-head posture. The last two positions are quite similar in the occiput-atlas relationship and the effect on how the teeth meet (occlusion). Most people find that their teeth touch in different places in the different head positions.

a. Based on this exercise, describe the association between head position and occlusion. Record the relationship of your teeth in each of the positions (e.g., lower teeth forward of regular bite).

b. Why might this occur? (You will need to know the myology of the TMJ to answer this.)

c. Management of TMJ dysfunction includes physical therapy and dental techniques. The dental techniques are often intended to change the patient's occlusion (bite). How should PT (physical therapy) and dental intervention be sequenced?

ANSWERS TO TEMPOROMANDIBULAR JOINT

*1. Check your texts to find these structures and then have a faculty member confirm your palpations.

*2. Use this exercise to practice facial observation skills. You will probably find many examples of asymmetry. Mild asymmetry is the norm and is of no consequence functionally. You may find some examples of marked asymmetry that are still of no functional consequence. You may also find some deviations that could be functionally significant. Have a faculty member confirm your observations.

*3. Make sure that you demonstrate, see, and feel the two distinct motions involved in mouth opening.

*4. Use this exercise to practice your palpation skills. You may find several examples of asymmetrical movement and popping or clicking.

5. No lateral deviation is usually seen during mouth opening and closing in an individual with a normal TMJ. Many instances of lateral deviation do occur, however. They are often totally asymptomatic and should not be treated.

6. When one articulation is affected by anything, the other articulation will also be affected. Since the connection between the two articulations is rigid (the mandible), any stress or force on one joint will be transmitted in some manner to the other joint.

7. Medially and laterally, the disc is attached firmly to the poles of the condyle of the mandible; there are no medial or lateral attachments of the disc to the capsule. The anterior portion of the disc is attached to the capsule and the superior portion of the lateral pterygoid muscle. The posterior aspect of the disc is attached to the bilaminar retrodiscal pad. This pad is composed of two bands. One band is attached to the tympanic plate through elastic fibers; the other band is attached to the neck of the condyle and is not elastic.

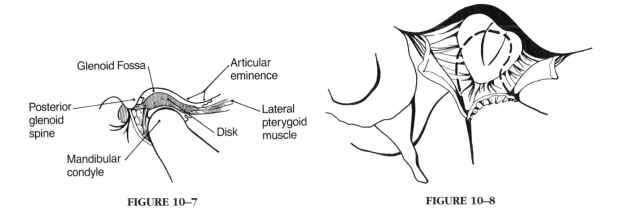

FIGURE 10–7

FIGURE 10–8

8. During normal mouth opening, the disc rotates posteriorly on the condyle during the rotation phase of the motion and then glides forward with the condyle during the translation phase of the motion. On closure, the process is reversed. First the disc and condyle glide posteriorly, and then the disc rotates anteriorly over the condyle to return to the initial closed-mouth position.

*9. A person can typically place the width of three of his own PIP joints between the upper and lower teeth. An opening of two PIP joints is functional. This measurement is too gross for specific evaluation of TMJ function, but it can be an effective home assessment for the patient.

   The most common method of measuring joint motion is by using a ruler to measure the motion (in millimeters) in each direction. Generally accepted ranges of motion are:

   40 to 50 mm of opening
   8 mm of lateral deviation to each side
   6 to 9 mm of protrusion
   3 mm of retrusion (note that this movement is not often measured)

*10. Use this exercise to practice observational skills. Have a faculty member confirm your observations.

*11. Have a faculty member confirm your palpations.

12–16. The completed outlines were provided in the myology section of the workbook.

17. During the rotation phase of normal mouth opening, the disc is restrained by the posterior attachments of the disc, which causes a posterior rotation of the disc in relation to the condyle. During the translation phase of mouth opening, the disc moves forward with the condyle by virtue of its firm attachments to the condylar poles. The inferior lamina of the retrodiscal pad limits forward excursion of the disc. See Figures 10-7 and 10-8 in the answer to item 7 (page 173).

   During mouth closing, the disc is pulled posteriorly by the elastic fibers of the superior lamina of the retrodiscal pad. The superior portions of the lateral pterygoid muscles contract eccentrically to control the posterior motion of the disc.

*18. A posteriorly dislocated disc limits mandibular elevation (mouth closing) by providing a mechanical block posterior to the condyle that does not allow the condyle to assume its normal position in the joint space. An anteriorly dislocated disc, on the other hand, limits mandibular depression (mouth opening) by not allowing the condyle to slide into a fully opened position. The rotation component is permitted, but the translation component is not complete.

*19. If only rotation is allowed to occur on the left, as the person begins opening the mouth, normal symmetrical motion occurs until the rotation phase is complete. As the person tries to continue opening the mouth, translation will occur on the right but will be unavailable on the left, causing the mandible to deviate to the left. This occurs because translation is continuing on the right, but no motion is occurring on the left. Make sure you re-create this motion using a skull and mandible. See Figure 10-9.

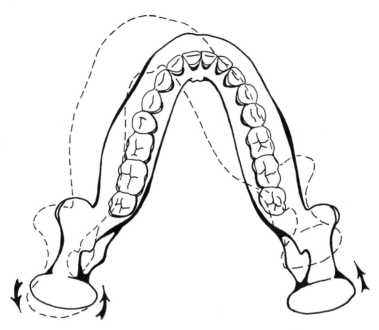

FIGURE 10–9

*20. The tight capsule limiting translation would create the same clinical picture as described in item 19. On mouth opening, Julia would have a C-curve to the left.

   Louis's motion, however, would be uneven. At first, on opening, his motion would be symmetrical. At the end of rotation, the mandible would deviate to the left as the disc limited translation on the left and translation occurred on the right. At the point when the disc would reduce (or relocate), the mandible would "jump" back to the midline as the translation on the left would be completed. On closure, the movement would also be uneven. As closure started, the movement would be even until the disc dislocated. At that point, the mandible would deviate to the left until the normal translation on the right was completed. As the translation on the right is completed, the mandible would be returning to the midline. The rotation phase of closing would probably be symmetrical. Individual variations from this general description are determined by tightness or looseness of the joint capsule and ligaments.

   In summary, a tight joint capsule creates a C-curve to the same side, while a dislocated disc creates a complex curve. Make sure you re-create these motions using a skull and mandible to gain a fuller understanding of the mechanism of the joint.

21. a. During extension of the head on the neck, the mandible tends to retract (move posteriorly in relation to the maxilla). During flexion, the mandible tends to protrude (move anteriorly in relation to the maxilla).

   b. This could be caused by tight musculature or soft-tissue impingement. For instance, extension of the head on the neck would tend to stretch the digastric, which would tend to retract the mandible. On the other hand, in extreme flexion of the head and neck, the soft tissues of the neck tend to push the mandible into a more protruded position.

   c. A forward-head posture is often present in a person with TMJ dysfunction. Physical therapy procedures are designed to affect posture, muscle length, strength, and coordination. These procedures often affect (decrease) the forward-head position of the patient. As this exercise has demonstrated, head position can affect occlusion (how the teeth come in contact with each other). Therefore, the physical therapist should see the patient early. If the PT is not involved in the case until after the dentist has completed work with the patient's occlusion, a great deal of dental work may need to be redone as the patient's occlusion changes through the PT treatments.

11 POSTURE

APPLICATIONS

Static posture results from the alignment of the body's segments so that the composite center of mass becomes vertically aligned over the base of support.

*1. On your laboratory partner, place colored stick-on markers on surface landmarks that will allow you to analyze her standing posture from the lateral and posterior views.

2. Describe the ideal standing posture of the body from a lateral and a posterior view.

3. You will be using a plumb line to examine the vertical relationship of the surface landmarks marked in item 1. To place the plumb line in a consistent manner among subjects, you need a consistent point of reference with which to align the plumb line. For this activity, you will be viewing posture from the lateral and posterior aspects; therefore, you will need a lateral and a posterior landmark for use as your point of reference for each view.

   Determine a logical point of reference for the lateral view and for the posterior view for your postural analysis.

*4. Compare the posture of five of your classmates with the ideal you described in item 2. Be sure to use the lateral and posterior views on each subject. In addition to the reference point landmark for the posterior view you chose in item 1, include the following bilateral assessments in your comparison:

Shoulder height   Gluteal folds
Orientation of scapula   Popliteal creases
Space between elbow and waist Medial malleoli
Height of iliac crests

5. What lines define the lumbosacral angle and what is the normal angle formed by those lines?

*6. Demonstrate an increased lumbosacral angle in the standing position.

7. Describe the posture of the hips and lumbar spine in the position you assumed in item 6. Use the Rule of Three.

*8. Demonstrate a decreased lumbosacral angle in the standing position.

9. Describe the posture of the hips and lumbar spine in the position you assumed in item 8. Use the Rule of Three.

*10. Examine normal posture from a lateral view using a plumb line and the landmarks you identified in item 1. From the normal standing position, place a 3-inch elevation under the subject's heels. What changes occur in the relationship of each landmark to the plumb line? Now place the elevation under the balls of the feet. What changes occur in the relationship of each landmark to the plumb line?

11. On Figure 11–1, assume the vertical line represents the line of gravity.

    a. What motion is the force of gravity attempting to produce at each lower extremity joint?

    b. What muscles at the hip and knee are responsible for counteracting the effect of gravity at each joint?

12. Assume the position drawn in Figure 11–1 and maintain it until you feel contraction in the hip and knee muscles responsible for maintaining the posture. Are they the same muscles you listed in item 11?

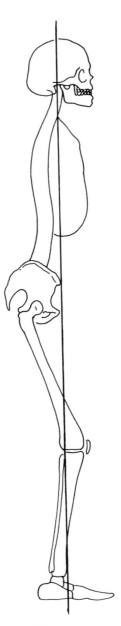

FIGURE 11–1

13. On Figure 11-2, assume that the vertical line represents the line of gravity.

   a. What is the effect of gravity at the hip and at the knee?

   b. Contrast the effect of gravity on the hip and the knee in Figures 11-1 and 11-2. Include a discussion of the relative magnitude of the effect as seen in each figure.

   c. Which posture requires greater energy to maintain?

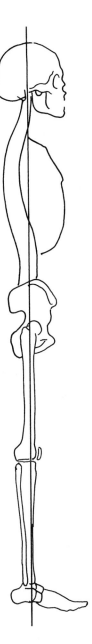

FIGURE 11–2

14. Given that the primary and secondary curves of the spine act as shock absorbers for vertical compression of the spine, what effect will decreasing the lumbosacral angle have on the shock absorption capacity of the lumbar spine?

*15. Have your partner sit in a chair and be sure that she assumes a relaxed position. Describe her lumbosacral angle in this sitting position.

*16. Do what you need to do to bring her lumbosacral angle in sitting back to a normal angle. Once you have corrected the lumbosacral angle, provide her with sufficient support so that she can relax and maintain the angle while sitting. State what you did to affect the angle.

17. While standing, assume a forward-head posture. Have a classmate verify the posture. What criteria did you use to determine what the posture would look like?

*18. Have your partner, in the sitting position, assume a pronounced forward-head posture. Now, have her raise her sternum. To do this, she will need to imagine that a vertical string is pulling her sternum up toward the ceiling. You should see her ribs rise as her sternum elevates. What effect did raising the sternum have on the forward-head posture? Would this work in a standing position?

*19. Have your partner stand in a posture as close to ideal as possible. Observe her spinal curves from the lateral view. Now, have her stand with a forward-head posture and note the spinal curves. Describe what you saw.

20. Explain how the forward-head posture places both sternocleidomastoid muscles in a shortened position.

21. On Figure 11–3, place a force vector representing the effect of gravity on the head. Note that the vertical line no longer represents the line of gravity; it is simply a reference point from which to judge posture. What deviations from ideal posture do you note in the illustration?

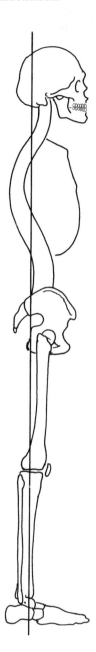

FIGURE 11–3

22. Complete the following table for Figure 11-3.

Joint to Assess	Anatomical Position of the Joint	Status of Muscles (shortened/lengthened) (indicate muscle and status)
Head on neck		
Cervical spine		
Cervical spine on thorax		
Thoracic spine		
Lumbar spine		
Pelvis		
Hip		
Knee		
Ankle		

*23. The weight of the human head is between 10 and 15 pounds. Hold a 10-pound weight in your hand and rest your elbow on the table with your forearm vertical. Extend your wrist with the weight resting in your open palm. Hold this position for 2 minutes. At the end of the 2 minutes, describe the sensation you feel in your wrist.

24. Explain the result of item 23 in terms of both the torque produced by gravity on the weight in your hand and the effort of the muscles responsible for counteracting that torque.

25. Relate items 21, 23, and 24.

26. Name the curves in the scolioses illustrated in Figures 11-4 and 11-5.

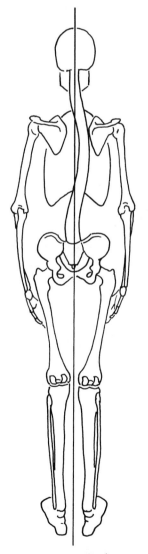

FIGURE 11–4

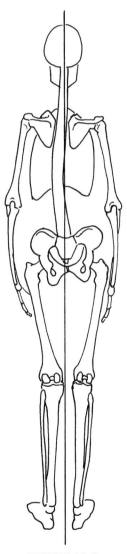

FIGURE 11–5

27. Complete the following table for Figure 11–5.

Joint to Assess	Anatomical Position of the Joint	Status of Muscles (shortened/lengthened) (indicate muscle and status)
Head		
Cervical spine		
Shoulders		
Thoracic spine		
Lumbar spine		
Pelvis		
Hips		
Knees		
Ankles		

*28. Place a dot over the spinous processes of all the palpable vertebrae on your partner. From a posterior view, evaluate the spine for deviations from vertical alignment. Have your partner bend forward. Does the alignment change in any way? Evaluate for scoliosis or rib humps. What view would you use to evaluate for kyphosis or flattening of the primary or secondary curves?

*29. Have your partner stand with a 1-inch elevation under the right foot, keeping both knees fully extended. From a posterior view, evaluate how this alters her posture.

30. For the purpose of this question and for scoliosis screening, assume that the thoracic vertebrae have coupled motion in the same pattern as the lumbar spine.
   a. What direction will the thoracic vertebrae rotate with right lateral bending of the thoracic spine?
   b. Which direction will the spinous processes move in conjunction with that vertebral rotation?
   c. If the right lateral bend is fixed, as in structural scoliosis, on which side will the posterior rib hump be noticed? Explain.

*31. In a public place, observe the posture of an individual who has a protruding abdomen, for example, a pregnant woman. Describe how this affects the individual's standing posture. Determine how this would affect the muscles responsible for maintaining the erect posture.

*32. Have your partner lie supine on a table and have her try to make one leg look longer than the other. What motion did she perform to accomplish this miraculous feat? Devise a measurement scheme to determine whether the leg is actually longer or some other explanation of this phenomenon exists.

*33. Measure segmental versus total leg length. What landmarks did you use to measure each segment? Discuss the reason for measuring both total length and segmental length, and a possible difficulty with using only one of those measurements.

ANSWERS TO POSTURE

*1. Your kinesiology text will probably show a lateral and posterior view of standing posture with a vertical line of gravity passing through the center of mass. Body landmarks typically used to examine posture will be named and located in relation to the vertical line. Some standard surface landmarks for the lateral view are the ear, acromion, greater trochanter, knee, and lateral malleolus. Landmarks for the posterior view are the nuchal eminence, spinous process of C-7, gluteal cleft, and midpoint between the feet.

2. In the ideal posture of the human body, the line of gravity falls close to most joint axes. The body segments are in near-vertical alignment; the compression forces are optimally distributed over weight-bearing surfaces. In particular, in a lateral view the line of gravity falls with the following relationships to joints and landmarks:

Slightly anterior to axis for flexion and extension of the head on the neck and through the external auditory meatus

Posterior to the lordotic curve of the cervical spine

Along the lateral border of the trunk (anterior to the kyphotic curve of the thoracic spine; posterior to the lordotic curve of the lumbar spine)

Slightly posterior to the axis of flexion and extension of the hip and roughly through the greater trochanter

Slightly anterior to the axis for flexion and extension of the knee

Slightly anterior to the axis for dorsiflexion and plantarflexion of the ankle and slightly anterior to the lateral malleolus

From a posterior view: The line of gravity will ideally bisect the body into left and right halves following the spinous processes and falling from the nuchal eminence through the gluteal cleft and arriving on the floor halfway between the feet.

3. The most typical landmark for consistent placement of the plumb line for a lateral assessment of posture is just anterior to the lateral malleolus. In a posterior view, either the nuchal eminence or a midposition between the heels can be used. A strong argument can be made for the feet as the landmark of choice because of their stability; however, Figure 11–5 uses the nuchal eminence. Once the plumb line has been placed over either of these landmarks, the remaining surface landmarks are examined with respect to where they fall in relation to the vertical line.

*4. This exercise allows you to appreciate the range of normal as well as assess classmates who may fall outside the range of normal. Frequently, a student is identified with a postural defect that had not been previously identified. This can be an uncomfortable situation that may need faculty input and supervision.

When you are examining the posterior view, the additional items listed allow for examination of symmetry between sides of the body in the frontal plane.

5. The lumbosacral angle is the angle formed by a line drawn parallel with the ground and another line drawn parallel to the superior plateau of the first sacral vertebra in the lateral view. The normal angle is about 30°.

*6. An increase in the lumbosacral angle is caused by anterior tilting of the sacrum (pelvis).

7. Flexion of the pelvis at the hip and an increase in anterior lumbar convexity (increased lumbar lordosis).

*8. A decreased lumbosacral angle is produced by a posterior pelvic tilt.

9. Extension of the pelvis at the hip and a decrease in the anterior lumbar convexity (decreased lumbar lordosis).

*10. The 3-inch elevation under the heels tends to cause the landmarks to move anteriorly. This anteriorly displaces the center of mass and thus anteriorly displaces the line of gravity in relation to the base of support. You should see the subject make an effort to move the center of mass posteriorly by increasing the lumbar lordosis and/or flexing the knees. When the elevation is placed under the toes, the reverse takes place. You may see the hips flex or some other effort to anteriorly displace the center of mass.

11. a. Hip and knee flexion; ankle dorsiflexion
    b. The hip extensors (gluteus maximus and hamstrings) are most responsible for resisting the force of gravity at the hip; the quadriceps are responsible for resisting the force of gravity at the knee.

*12. Sense the tension in the muscles listed in item 11.

13. a. Item 11 illustrates gravity producing a flexor moment at the hip and knee, whereas Figure 11–2 demonstrates the line of gravity falling slightly behind the axis for flexion and extension of the hip and slightly in front of the axis for flexion and extension of the knee. This alignment produces an extensor moment at each joint. The line of gravity falls farther away from the joint in item 11 (Figure 11–1) than in Figure 11–2, making the moment arm of the gravity force greater in item 11. With the greater moment arm and equivalent force, the torque in item 11 is greater than in item 13.

b. The combination of less torque and the turning moment being toward the stability of each joint makes the effort to maintain the posture in Figure 11–2 much less than the posture in Figure 11–1.

14. When the lumbosacral angle is decreased, more force from the weight of the upper body mass is transmitted directly to the vertebral bodies and intervertebral disks causing increased compression. Normally, the force is dissipated by the lumbar curve.

*15. The typical lumbosacral angle in sitting is decreased because the sacrum is more posteriorly tilted.

*16. You will probably provide some support for the posterior lumbar spine so that the normal lordotic curve reappears. The position will allow your partner to sit erect but relaxed.

*17. The simplest criterion is relative placement of the head on the neck, which is effectively assessed by the position of the zygomatic arch (cheekbone) over the manubrium. The commonly used alignment of the auditory canal over the acromion can be misleading if the individual has both a forward head and rounded shoulders. The rounding of the shoulders may place the acromion under the external auditory meatus, even with the forward-head posture.

*18. Raising the sternum typically reduces the forward-head posture. Yes, it will also apply in the standing position.

*19. Jutting the head forward increases the kyphotic posture of the thoracic spine and may increase or decrease the lordotic posture of the lumbar spine. The cervical spine shows flexion in the lower segments and extension in the upper segments.

20. The forward-head posture consists of extension of the head on the atlas and flexion of the lower cervical spine on the thorax. The sternocleidomastoid (SCM) muscle crosses posterior to the axis for flexion and extension of the head on the atlas and anterior to the axis for flexion and extension of the lower cervical spine on the thorax. Therefore, the forward-head posture shortens the SCM for both the head-on-atlas position and the lower cervical spine-on-thorax position.

21. Deviations from ideal posture include kyphosis and forward head.

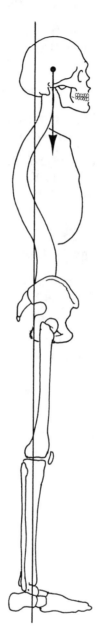

FIGURE 11–6

22. This is the completed table for Figure 11-3.

Joint to Assess	Anatomical Position of the Joint	Status of Muscles (shortened/lengthened) (indicate muscle and status)
Head on neck	Extended	Extensors—shortened Flexors—lengthened
Cervical spine	Increased lordosis	Extensors—shortened Flexors—lengthened
Cervical spine on thorax	Flexion	Extensors—lengthened Flexors—shortened
Thoracic spine	Increased kyphosis	Extensors—lengthened Flexors—shortened
Lumbar spine	Increased lordosis	Extensors—shortened Flexors—lengthened
Pelvis	Neutral on hip, but extended on lumbar spine	Lumbar extensors—shortened Abdominals—lengthened
Hip	Neutral	Balanced
Knee	Neutral	Balanced
Ankle	Increased dorsiflexion	Soleus—lengthened Dorsiflexors—shortened

*23. You will probably feel a sense of overstretching and fatigue in the muscles controlling the wrist.

24. The force of gravity falls posterior to the axis for flexion and extension producing an extension moment at the wrist. The wrist flexors attempt to counterbalance this torque, but in a mechanically disadvantageous position.

25. Fatigue and strain can occur in the posterior muscles of the neck and upper back when they are required to maintain the head upright against a flexion moment of the force of gravity, as in item 21. This is analogous to the result in the wrist in items 23 and 24.

26. The scoliosis diagrams demonstrate a left lumbar, right thoracic curve (Figure 11–4) and a left thoracolumbar curve (Figure 11–5).

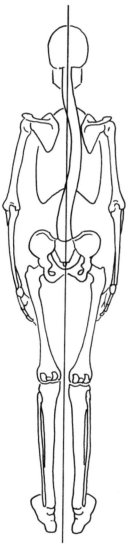

FIGURE 11–4

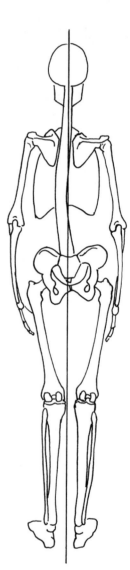

FIGURE 11–5

27. This is the completed table for Figure 11-5.

Joint to Assess	Anatomical Position of the Joint	Status of Muscles (shortened/lengthened) (indicate muscle and status)
Head	Neutral	Balanced
Cervical spine	Head to right of lower C-spine	Right lateral mm—lengthened Left lateral mm—shortened
Shoulders	Left—high Right—low	Right upper trapezius—lengthened Left upper trapezius—shortened
Thoracic spine	Left thoracic C-curve (convexity to the left)	Right lateral trunk mm—shortened Left lateral trunk mm—lengthened
Lumbar spine	Left lumbar C-curve (convexity to the left)	Right lateral trunk mm—shortened Left lateral trunk mm—lengthened
Pelvis	Right side of pelvis is elevated	Right hip elevators—lenghtened Left hip elevators—shortened (The figure shows a decrease in the angle between the left pelvis and the lumbar spine, which is reflected in this answer. If there were no scoliosis, and the pelvis was laterally tilted, this answer would not be correct.)
Hips	Right hip—adducted Left hip—abducted	Right lateral hip mm—lengthened Right medial hip mm—shortened Left lateral hip mm—shortened Left medial hip mm—lengthened
Knees	Neutral	Balanced
Ankles	Mild pronation bilaterally	Supinators—lengthened Pronators—shortened

* 28. Often, if a subject shows a mild lateral curve in standing, it will disappear in forward bending, indicating that it is a functional (not fixed) curve. If the curve remains on forward bending, it is considered to be structural (fixed). The lateral view is necessary to see changes in the primary and secondary curves.

* 29. A unilateral lift under the right foot with the right knee straight transmits the effect of the elevation directly to the lumbosacral junction. The pelvis will tip laterally, the right iliac crest will be higher than the left, and you may see a left lumbar curve in the spine. This exercise simulates the effect of the right leg being longer than the left when the subject is standing with bilateral knees extended.

30. a. Right lateral bend in the thoracic spine produces left rotation of the vertebrae.
    b. With left rotation of the vertebrae, you observe movement of the spinous processes to the right.
    c. The ribs will follow the vertebrae, so the right ribs will move forward and the left ribs will move back as the vertebrae rotate to the left. If the right lateral bend is fixed as in a structural scoliosis, there will be a posterior rib hump on the left because the curve of the left ribs has moved back and become fixed with the fixed vertebrae.

* 31. A disproportionate amount of weight placed anteriorly to the normal center of mass will cause a compensatory posterior displacement of the upper trunk. This adjustment is most obvious in the lumbar spine. To maintain this posture, the lumbar spinal extensors may be overactive.

* 32. This movement is accomplished by lateral tipping of the pelvis. Most of your patients, however, will not try to make one leg longer than the other. To determine whether one leg is longer than the other, or whether the pelvis is tipped, you must compare the measurements of both the bony length of the leg and the length from the midline of the trunk (usually the navel). Differences in leg length demonstrated by the measurement from the midline of the trunk may be due to lateral tipping of the pelvis, since the tipping will move the leg with the pelvis. Measurements of the length of the leg itself, from the anterior superior iliac spine (ASIS) to the medial malleolus, are not affected by pelvic tipping. Therefore, differences in the leg length measured from the ASIS to the medial malleolus would demonstrate actual bone length differences.

* 33. You should be able to pick proximal and distal bony landmarks on the thigh and on the lower leg to use to measure each bone. When a short leg is noted, measuring segmentally allows you to determine which bone is short. However, segmental measuring can increase the error in the measurement. Total leg length measured from ASIS to medial malleolus is better for eliminating errors, but determining the involved bone or segment is more difficult.

    If a short leg is found, two screening techniques can assist in determining the short segment of the lower limb. The principle behind these two test positions is to place the respective rigid lever (femur or tibia) between the knee and supporting surface.

    First, assess the knee height with the subject supine and hips flexed to 90° (feet off the table, knees flexed). This can give a visual estimate of comparative femur length. This assumes that there are no significant pelvic anomalies and that the pelvis is not unduly rotated on the lumbar spine.

    Next, assess knee height with the subject supine, hips and knees flexed, and both feet together and flat on the examining table. This will give a visual estimate of comparative tibial length, as the tibia are now supporting the height of the knee.

12 GAIT
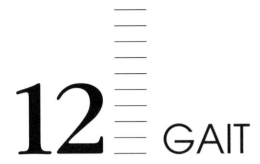

PHASES OF GAIT

Gait and ambulation are the terms used for human locomotion. The normal gait pattern is divided into two phases.

1. Name the two phases of gait.

2. The subdivisions of each gait cycle have been described using various terms. The two most common terminology systems are the traditional (more standard) and the newer Rancho Los Amigos (RLA) systems. Using the lists below, match the standard terminology of gait with the RLA terminology for gait. Throughout this chapter, we will be using RLA terminology.

Traditional	**Traditional**	**RLA**	**RLA**
Heel strike	Acceleration	Terminal swing	Loading response
Toe-off	Deceleration	Preswing	Midswing
Foot flat	Midstance	Initial contact	Terminal stance
Heel-off	Midswing	Initial swing	Midstance

3. On Figure 12-1, label each subdivision of the phases of gait for the *right lower extremity* using the RLA nomenclature.

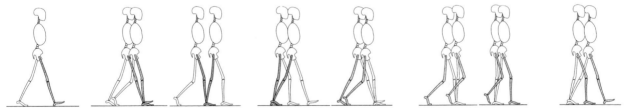

FIGURE 12–1. From Perry J: Gait Analysis: Normal and Pathological Function. Slack Incorporated, Thorofare, New Jersey, 1992, pp 12-15, with permission.

4. Give the movement occurring in the noted joints within each subdivision of gait. If the box is occupied with XXX, ignore that joint's movement.

Joint	Initial Contact and Loading Response	Midstance	Terminal Stance	Preswing	Initial Swing	Midswing	Terminal Swing
Hip	XXX						XXX
Knee			XXX				
Ankle			XXX				XXX

5. Describe the movement of the shoulder girdle and upper extremities in concert with the lower extremities.

6. Considering the right lower extremity, at which subdivisions of the gait cycle does each of the two periods of double support occur?

7. At which part(s) of the gait cycle is the knee in maximal flexion?

DISTANCE AND TIME VARIABLES

8. How is stride length determined?

9. Contrast stride length and step length.

10. How is the velocity of gait determined?

11. Discuss the relationship between cadence and length of the period of double support.

*12. Ask a subject to stand without moving on a large piece of paper. Draw an outline of the base of support in standing. Now, have the subject mimic midstance. Draw an outline of the base of support during midstance. Finally, have the subject mimic the position during double-limb support (R—initial contact/loading response and L—preswing). Draw an outline of the base of support during double-limb support. How did you determine the size and shape of each drawing?

13. Compare the differences in distance between medial malleoli during gait between a young child and a young adult and between a young adult and an elderly adult. To what do you attribute the differences? (Note: If there is no easy reference from which to create your description, use observation of the public in an area such as a shopping plaza or theater.)

14. What is the normal degree of toe-out during gait?

   a. How does the normal degree of toe-out change with increased speed of gait?

   b. How does the degree of toe-out relate to the size of the base of support?

   c. How does the size of the base of support relate to static stability?

   d. What is the relationship of static stability to mobility?

   e. What is a possible function of the change in degree of toe-out with increased speed?

*15. For this activity you will need powder, a carpeted surface for walking, a chair, a long string, a goniometer, and a ruler. In a sitting position with your feet dangling, place powder on the plantar surface of your bare feet. Then stand up with your feet a comfortable distance apart. From this position, walk through at least two full gait cycles on the carpeted surface. Come to a complete stop on the last cycle.

   a. Using a line between the medial borders of consecutive right-heel prints, measure the degree of right toe-out during ambulation versus the degree of toe-out when you came to a standing position. How can you account for the difference in degrees, if there was a difference?

   b. Measure the stride length and step width.

DETERMINANTS OF GAIT

*16. Standing behind a partner, lightly place your hands on both sides of his pelvis (iliac crests). Have your partner walk while you continue to feel the movement of the pelvis during ambulation. Make sure you do not inhibit your partner's normal gait motion. Describe the movements of the pelvis during gait.

*17. Repeat item 16, but have your partner walk with the feet close together (decreased medial and lateral base of support), then with the feet spread far apart. How does this affect the movement of the pelvis? Describe how this affects the relationship of the center of gravity and the base of support.

* 18. Demonstrate how pelvic rotation in the horizontal plane over the stationary femur on the stance limb effectively lengthens the swinging limb. You can accomplish this by consciously avoiding any pelvic rotation during gait, then allowing it and observing the difference in stride of the swing limb. Remember that the pelvic rotation is occurring in the stance hip.

19. How does the normal pelvic rotation described in item 18 affect the energy requirement of gait?

20. Explain how movement of the center of gravity during gait affects the expenditure of energy associated with gait.

21. Explain how lack of knee flexion can increase the energy cost of gait.

22. During stance, the pelvis drops slightly toward the unsupported side. The interaction of pelvic drop with knee extension at midstance decreases the energy cost of ambulation. Explain.

23. The angle of inclination of the femoral neck on the shaft was discussed in Chapter 4. What effect does this angle have on the base of support in the standing position?

24. What angle at the knee compensates for the effect of the femoral angle of inclination, thus preventing the feet from crossing each other in the standing position?

25. The interaction of knee and ankle motion during gait tends to shorten the *stance* limb from initial contact to midstance and tends to lengthen it relatively from midstance to preswing. What is the effect of this on the movement of the center of mass during stance?

26. Based on items 18 to 25, what are the six determinants of gait?

27. Why are the determinants of gait important for efficient ambulation?

MYOLOGY OF GAIT

28. During which subdivision of gait are the dorsiflexors of the ankle most active? Hint: For the myology questions, review the grid completed for question 4.

    a. What type of contraction are they performing?

    b. What is the function of this contraction?

29. The gastrocnemius-soleus complex is quite active during midstance.
    a. What joint motion at the ankle is occurring during midstance?

    b. What is the function of this contraction of the gastrocnemius–soleus group?

    c. What type of contraction is it?

30. Why is a contraction of the quadriceps necessary at initial contact/loading response?

31. Explain why the hamstrings are active during both terminal swing and initial contact.

32. What is the function of the gluteus maximus in the early stance phase of gait?

33. During which subdivision of gait are the hip flexors most active? What function are they performing?

34. What is the function of the abductor muscles of the stance hip during initial contact/loading response? In what fashion do these muscles contract during initial contact through midstance?

35. In which subdivision of gait are the erector spinae muscles most active?

MOMENTUM

*36. a. Walk *very slowly* for about 20 ft. Think about how the muscles around your hips, knees, and ankles *feel*.
   b. Walk at a normal pace and think about how the muscles around your hips, knees, and ankles *feel*.
   c. Walk at normal speed. Stop suddenly on one foot. What happens to your body or balance? Think about how the muscles around your stance hip, knee, and ankle feel.
   d. What is an explanation of the difference in muscle activity you felt between a and b?

   e. Explain what happened to your body position or balance and what you felt in c.

f. What inferences concerning the role of momentum in normal gait can you make as a result of items a through e?

37. Item 36 demonstrates the value of momentum in maintaining forward propulsion in gait. Examine normal gait and identify which joint motions during gait are primarily caused by momentum. Identify as many sources of momentum as you can.

APPLICATIONS

*38. In groups of five, select two subjects in the group to walk so that the other group members can observe normal gait. The subjects should be in laboratory clothes.

a. Determine bony landmarks on which to apply markers to enhance the observation of joint motion in the sagittal and frontal planes. In making your choices, be sure to include markers that will allow you to view tibial and pelvic rotation in the horizontal plane and elevation and depression of the center of mass. Apply the markers. Hint: A soda straw taped so that it appears to penetrate the anterior tibia and a second penetrating the sacrum will accentuate the effect of tibial and pelvic rotation, making them much easier to observe.

b. Have one subject walk at a time so that all members get a chance to observe normal gait. The subject should walk normally at a moderate rate. Have the subject walk while the other members in the group record what is occurring at each joint during each subdivision of the gait cycle. Observers will find it most effective to focus on one joint at a time and to change the focus of observation in an orderly fashion, either from the foot up or from the head down.

c. Include in your description for b what motion is occurring at each joint during each subdivision of the gait cycle.

d. Observe the elevation and depression of the center of mass during gait. Determine at what subdivisions of the gait cycle the center of mass is highest and lowest.

*e. Stand with your left side next to a chalkboard. Hold a long piece of brightly colored chalk (yellow, for instance) so that it is at the level of your left shoulder and touches the board. Have your elbow bent so that your hand is touching your shoulder. For this exercise to work, you must be able to keep the chalk steady while you are walking. Now, with the chalk in contact with the board, walk at a normal speed parallel to the board. When you reach the other end of the board, stop and examine the chalk line. You will see a low-amplitude sinusoidal curve. Now walk with a stiff right knee using a different-colored chalk.

1. Measure the distance from the lowest to highest points on the curve.
2. At what point in the gait cycle is the highest point on the curve?
3. At what point in the gait cycle is the lowest point?
4. What change occurs in the curve on the board when you walk with a stiff right knee? What does that change suggest about a change in energy expenditure?

*39. Have a subject mimic severe weakness in the left gastrocnemius–soleus. The step length of which limb will be most affected by the weakness? Why?

40. At what other point of the gait cycle, in addition to loading response, will you easily be able to see the effect of a weak tibialis anterior?

41. What foot and ankle muscles can assist the action of a weak tibialis anterior?

42. Motion at what joints near the ankle will mask the effect of fusion of the talocrural joint?

*43. Demonstrate a gait pattern for each of the following muscle weaknesses:
    a. Bilateral gluteus maximus
    b. Unilateral gluteus medius
    c. Bilateral iliopsoas
    d. Unilateral quadriceps
    e. Unilateral pretibial group

*44. Use a low cart or board with wheels underneath (such as a scooter board) to examine Newton's three laws of motion. In the following examples, the scooter board becomes a barometer of applied force and the relative reactions to applied forces. The following activities are designed to demonstrate the three laws of motion. These activities are courtesy of Dr. D. Michael McKeough while he was Associate Professor in the Department of Physical Therapy, Medical College of Georgia.

NOTE: In our experience, these scooter-board activities have been best demonstrated by a faculty member with the students observing. The activity is then followed by class discussion. We have found the activities valuable in relating the laws of motion to gait. Care should be exercised in performing these activities.

a. Stand beside the scooter board and take a vigorous step forward. Look at your location after this step. Next, stand on the scooter board and take a vigorous step forward off the scooter board (expect the scooter board to move backward quickly). Compare your location at the end of each step. Compare the movement of your body and the movement of the scooter board. The movement of the scooter board (the second step), which has a much lower mass than the earth or your body, is significantly greater than the movement of your body (the first step). This is a demonstration of Newton's second law of motion. Explain this in your own words.

b. Place as many weights on the scooter board as you can and still have a place to stand. Now take a vigorous step off the board and note the distance it travels as opposed to the distance of your step. How do these distances compare to the distances seen in a? Write out the equation for Newton's second law of motion in terms of these two activities.

c. Take the weights off the scooter board. Stand on the scooter board and take a *normal* step off as you begin to walk away. Note the distance the scooter board moved. This distance is a reflection of the force needed to get you going from standing still. What law does this activity relate to?

d. Now, place the scooter board in a walkway and walk so that one of your feet steps squarely onto the scooter board during your walking. As you leave the board, note the distance it moves backward during normal gait. This distance reflects the force needed to maintain normal gait. In which case did the board move further back, c or d? Explain why the two distances are different.

*45. Since normal gait is a continuous series of anticipated responses, the ambulator is consistently counting on the reaction force of the ground to propel him. To demonstrate the effect of the ground reaction force working in concert with the coefficient of friction between the foot and the ground, walk straight ahead until you step squarely on the scooter board (as in item 44d above). Immediately make a 90° turn off the foot that is on the scooter board. For example, if you are on your right, turn to the left by pushing off the right. Be prepared for the scooter board to move suddenly and vigorously. The movement of the scooter board is an indicator for the ground reaction force and friction force needed to change directions.

a. Ground reaction force is an example of which of Newton's laws?
b. Do any other above activities relate to this same law?

46. During gait, momentum provides considerable force to sustain forward progression. To which of Newton's laws is momentum most directly related?

ANSWERS TO GAIT

1. The two phases of gait are swing and stance phase.

2. | **Traditional** | **RLA** |
   |---|---|
   | Heel strike | Initial contact |
   | Foot flat | Part of loading response |
   | Midstance | Part of midstance |
   | Heel-off | Part of terminal stance |
   | Toe-off | Preswing |
   | Acceleration | Part of initial swing and midswing |
   | Midswing | Part of midswing and terminal swing |
   | Deceleration | Part of terminal swing |

3. Correct labels for Figure 12–1.

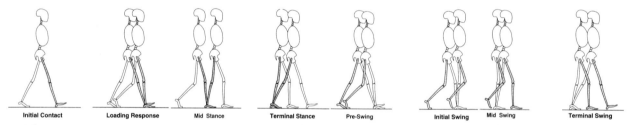

Initial Contact   Loading Response   Mid Stance   Terminal Stance   Pre-Swing   Initial Swing   Mid Swing   Terminal Swing

FIGURE 12–2. From Perry J: Gait Analysis: Normal and Pathological Function. Slack Incorporated, Thorofare, New Jersey, 1992, pp 12–15, with permission.

4. This is the completed table for Figure 12–1.

Joint	Initial Contact and Loading Response	Midstance	Terminal Stance	Preswing	Initial Swing	Midswing	Terminal Swing
Hip	XXX	extending	extending	flexing	flexing	flexing	XXX
Knee	flexing	extending	XXX	flexing	flexing	extending	extending
Ankle	plantar-flexing	dorsi-flexing	XXX	plantar-flexing	dorsi-flexing	dorsi-flexing	XXX

5. The upper-limb movement is in concert with the contralateral lower limb, for example, as the left lower limb moves forward, so does the right upper limb. This reciprocal relationship occurs with counterrotation between the shoulder and pelvic girdles.

6. Double support occurs at initial contact/loading response and again at preswing. These periods of double-limb support are the periods of greatest static stability, and as the speed of walking slows, the length of time in double support increases. Patients with decreased balance or stability naturally tend to walk more slowly.

7. The knee reaches its maximum degree of flexion between initial swing and midswing.

8. Stride length is determined by measuring the distance from the point of initial contact of one extremity to the next initial contact of the same extremity.

9. Stride length is measured in relation to the ipsilateral extremity, while step length is measured from initial contact of one extremity to initial contact of the other extremity.

10. The velocity of gait is determined by the number of steps completed per minute multiplied by the step length. This gives the distance covered per minute.

11. As cadence increases, the duration of double support decreases.

*12. The base of support is that area between and under both feet, if both feet are on the floor, or under one foot if it is on the floor alone as in midstance. Therefore, when both feet are on the ground, the drawing of the base of support will include the area between the feet as well as under the feet.

13. The width of the base of support in children is wider than in adults because of a higher center of gravity (COG) and decreased equilibrium reactions in children. An elderly adult also has a wider base of support than a younger adult because of the elderly adult's slower gait pattern and slowed reaction time, which require greater static stabilization.

14. There are 7° of normal toe-out during ambulation.
    a. As speed increases, the degree of toe-out decreases.
    b. The greater the degree of toe-out, the larger the area of the base of support.
    c. The larger the base of support, the greater the static stability.
    d. There is an inverse relationship between static stability and mobility. As one goes up, the other must go down.
    e. Increased speed requires increased mobility. Increased speed also provides dynamic stability, as in riding a bicycle. As the speed of ambulation increases, the requirement and usefulness of toe-out decrease.

*15. a. The line between successive heel impressions of the same foot is the reference line against which the angle of toe-out is measured. This is the line of progression. A midline is chosen on the powder footprint, and the goniometer is placed along it and the line of progression. This activity reinforces use of the goniometer and solves the problem of where the reference line is drawn in relation to the footprint.
    b. Horizontal lines will have to be drawn across the back of the heel prints in order to measure from one to the other. The horizontals will have to be parallel in order to measure from one foot to the other to obtain step length. This exercise leads to discussion of what effect certain gait abnormalities have on stride versus step length and why.
       Step width is the distance between parallel lines of progression, one for the right and one for the left.

*16. You should feel rotation in the horizontal plane, lateral tilting in the frontal plane, and a lateral shift from one foot to the other.

*17. As the feet become wider apart, the lateral shift will increase in order to get the center of gravity over the stance foot. This increases the lateral excursion of the center of gravity and the energy output.

*18. The rotating pelvis will bring the swinging hip forward, placing the foot farther in front.

19. The apparent lengthening of the lower limbs by the pelvic rotation serves to diminish the amount of drop of the center of mass for a given step length. In order to maintain the same step length but without pelvic rotation, the hips would have to flex and extend farther, producing a greater vertical excursion of the center of mass.

20. Vertical displacement of the center of gravity creates work and energy expenditure. Lateral movement of the center of gravity creates linear momentum that must be counteracted by muscular effort and thus creates an expenditure of energy.

21. Lack of knee flexion causes compensatory movements such as hip hiking on the affected side or circumducting the affected lower limb to clear the foot off the ground during swing phase. These compensations cause an increase in the vertical displacement of the center of gravity. Lack of knee flexion also disrupts the interaction between the ankle and the knee and the smooth transition to stance. All of this increases the energy cost of gait.

22. The extended stance limb at midstance tends to elevate the center of gravity. The pelvic drop allows the center of gravity to fall and compensates for the extended midstance limb which has raised the COG. The pelvic drop helps limit the excursion of the center of mass.

23. The angle of inclination, with the femoral head seated in the acetabulum, guides the shaft of the femur toward the midline, thus narrowing the base of support.

24. Physiological valgus at the knee.

25. The transition from swing to stance phase accompanies the transition from a descending to an ascending center of gravity. To smooth that transition, the knee flexes following initial contact and the foot plantar flexes from initial contact through loading response. This effectively shortens the limb as the center of gravity starts to rise, slowing the rise. The extension of the knee with plantar flexion of the ankle from midstance through preswing effectively does the reverse; that is, apparently lengthens the stance limb to decrease the descent of the center of gravity because it is now moving downward from its highest elevation at midstance.

26. The determinants of gait include: (1) pelvic rotation in the horizontal plane, (2) lateral pelvic tilt (drop to the unsupported side), (3) knee flexion, (4 and 5) knee with ankle interactions (shortening or lengthening a limb), and (6) physiologic valgus at the knee.

27. The determinants of gait help to minimize vertical rise of the COG, prevent an excessive drop in the body's COG, minimize the side-to-side movement of the COG, and provide a smooth transition to the weight-bearing limb, which smoothes the movement of the COG in space. All these effects serve to minimize energy expenditure during normal gait.

28. The dorsiflexors of the ankle are most active during initial contact and loading response.
    a. Eccentric
    b. Prevents the foot from slapping the ground in the transition from initial contact to loading response.

29. a. Dorsiflexion
    b. To slow the dorsiflexion or stabilize the ankle as the line of gravity passes in front of the ankle, producing a dorsiflexion moment.
    c. Eccentric because dorsiflexion is occurring.

30. At initial contact/loading response, the line of gravity and the line of force up the limb from the foot striking the ground fall behind the knee-joint axis, producing a flexion moment at the knee. The quadriceps contracts to prevent the knee from buckling.

31. The hamstrings function to decelerate the forward swing of the limb and to prevent excessive hip flexion as well as knee extension because of momentum. They also serve with the gluteus maximus to stabilize the hip at initial contact/loading response when the body weight is carried on a flexed hip.

32. The gluteus maximus provides hip control on the stance limb.

33. The hip flexors are most active during initial swing and are responsible for the initiation of the swing phase of gait.

34. The abductor muscles function as lateral stabilizers of the pelvis, preventing excessive lowering of the pelvis on the unsupported side during the stance phase of gait. As the pelvis drops, the contraction is eccentric. While the pelvis is stable, the contraction is isometric.

35. The erector spinae muscles are most active during initial contact/loading response. The right erector spinae contract when the right heel strikes the ground, and contract again, but more strongly, when the left heel hits the ground. Because the left erector spinae are performing the reverse of the right, both contract at each initial contact, but asymmetrically, depending on which heel is hitting the ground.

* 36. d. The muscles of gait contract almost continuously when you walk slowly because there is no dynamic balance or momentum to keep you up or moving.
   e. Normal gait is propelled to a great extent by momentum (inertia). This force keeps you going if you try to stop quickly.
   f. Once the body is moving, short bursts of muscle contraction keep it going. The tendency to fall forward if you stop quickly is a barometer of the force of momentum in gait.

37. The joint motions relying on momentum are the completion of flexion of the humerus at the shoulder, completion of flexion of the femur at the hip in swing phase, extension of the tibia at the knee in swing phase, extension of the femur at the hip in stance phase, completion of extension of the tibia at the knee in stance phase, dorsiflexion of the tibia at the ankle in stance phase. There are at least two sources of momentum: the swinging limbs, primarily the lower limb, and the push-off of the gastrocnemius soleus from terminal stance through preswing.

* 38. a. Concentrate on placement of the markers around major joints and on parts having wide excursions of movement. Using trial and error a few times will help you decide the best locations to assist observation. The two exceptions are to place markers on the crest of the tibia and on the sacrum so that rotation of the tibia and pelvis in the horizontal plane can be observed.
     To evaluate vertical displacement of the center of mass, use a marker on the trunk lateral to the location of the center of mass.
   c. Actions of the joints can be confirmed by your kinesiology text.
   d. The COG is at its highest at midstance and lowest at double-limb support.
   e. 1. The distance from the lowest to highest points on the sinusoidal curve should not be more than 2 inches. Why?
      2. Midstance
      3. Double limb support
      4. The curve is higher at left midstance in order to help clear the right foot during right swing. The energy expenditure will increase because the vertical excursion of the COG (work) increases.

* 39. Right step length will be shortened because stance on the left will be prematurely terminated. In order to extend stance on the left, the gastrocnemius-soleus must stabilize the ankle when the line of gravity falls anterior to the joint. This occurs during midstance, when the swing leg is moving toward terminal swing.

40. Weakness of the tibialis anterior also causes a "steppage gait" during swing phase. In order to clear the toes from the ground, the individual will lift the knee higher than normal, using increased hip flexion and possibly increased knee flexion.

41. Other muscles available to assist the tibialis anterior are the other anterior compartment muscles, the extensor digitorum longus, and the extensor hallucis longus.

42. The midtarsal and tarsometatarsal joints can mask a fused talocrural joint.

* 43. a. Posterior trunk lurch bilaterally to keep the line of gravity well posterior to the hip
   b. Lateral trunk lurch over the stance hip
   c. Forward thrust of the pelvis at each initial swing
   d. Genu recurvatum at initial contact/loading response or press the knee into locked extension with the ipsilateral hand
   e. Steppage during swing and foot slap at initial contact/loading response
   Demonstration or confirmation by a faculty member is helpful in this activity.

* 44. These four activities are self-explained within the context of the item. Review of the three laws of motion assists the discussion and aids further discussion of how each activity can reflect aspects of each of the laws other than the highlighted one. The activities aid the discussion of the contribution of momentum to the force of locomotion and discussion of the relative force of propulsion of the hip extensors and plantarflexors when overcoming static inertia.

* 45. This activity dramatically demonstrates the contribution of the resistance of the ground to the direction and continuation of locomotion. An appreciation should develop that, in moving forward or when turning, the body's effort is in a posterior or lateral direction and that it is actually the returned force of the ground that propels the body in the opposite direction.

    a. This is an example of the third law, the Law of Reaction.
    b. While items 44a, b, and c most directly apply to the Law of Acceleration (the second law), they can also be seen as applications of the third law.

  46. The law of inertia.